Silenced

Samantha Maxwell

ISBN 9798264502163

Wordworx
Wrexham Enterprise Hub
11-13 Rhosddu Road Wrexham
LL11 1AT

Silenced

Samantha Maxwell

Favourite Quotes I Personally Live By

"If you enter this world knowing you are loved and you leave this world knowing the same, then everything that happens in between can be dealt with." – [Michael Jackson]

"In complete darkness we are all the same, it is only our knowledge and wisdom that separates us, don't let your eyes deceive you." – [Janet Jackson, Livin' In Complete Darkness, Janet Jackson's Rhythm Nation 1814, 1989]

Two of my favourite quotes which are not only thought provoking, but are also true. You can adapt these quotes to any subject regarding society, and they make complete sense. – Samantha

Dedicated to my lovely family, who supported me during my own mental health deterioration.
Thank you so much.

I love you all.

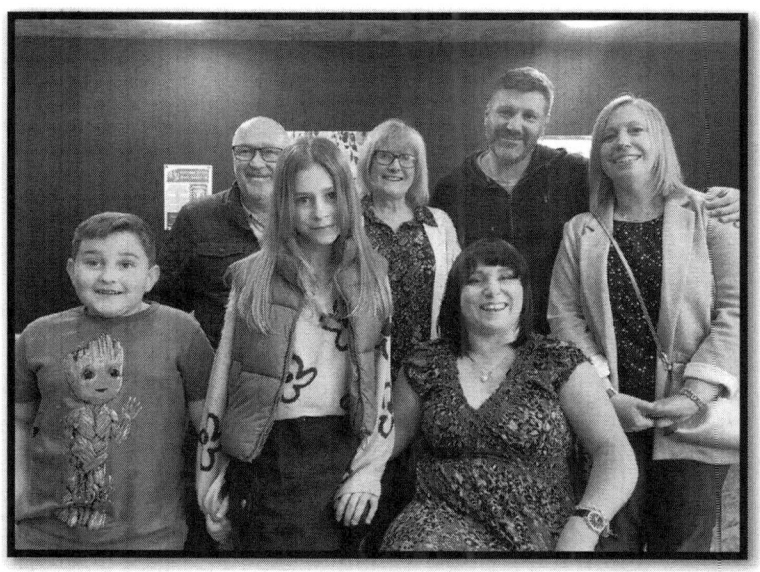

Foreword

Life is all fun and games until you develop a mental health issue of some kind. Then people around you, it seems, tend to fall into one of two camps, fight or flee. It's this mentality that can either make or break a person further who is suffering, or indeed help them through. The situation we find ourselves in, can play a massive part in how we deal with those challenges and insecurities. Things which can have a damaging effect on us mentally if not recognised and treated sooner. A whole host of different factors could be the reason for mental health decline, but for the purposes of this book, the subject matter is going to delve into the disability side of mental health.

Disability is a stigma all on its own. The term tends to bring with it a whole host of unnecessary challenges such as patronisation, discrimination, segregation etc. General society cannot seem to understand or are actually interested that disability is mistreated. Often, a person with a disability is left alone, isolated, in a physical, mental and emotional sense, because this mentality of 'disability is equal to difference' has unfortunately been ingrained into society over the years.

Ideally, we all need people around us. Human beings are social creatures by nature, regardless of who we are as an individual, and this need isn't as crucial as when a mental health issue develops. Now, not to downplay life by saying that it's all fun and games, because of course it isn't. You must work hard if you want to achieve your goals. Never more so it seems then when you have a disability of some form. The cards are automatically stacked against you, but nothing worth having, ever comes easy, which really, in all honesty, if you're talking specifically about general society, are all everyday stresses of life, which, in turn, may have a knock-on affect to our mental health, and so others may choose to distance themselves away from the person as they may not want any added stress or worry.

Life is fast paced and stressful as it is, without adding the stress of others on top. People may choose to distance themselves away from a person with a mental health issue, and so, people may look for others as a replacement, somebody that isn't 'stressed'. Somebody who is 'easier' to befriend. This is where the isolation factor comes into play for the person with a mental health issue, as they maybe left alone until they 'snap out of it'. This terminology only exasperates an already fragile issue, with extreme consequences sometimes. The truth is that the whole world is undoubtedly stressed at some point in their lives. It's just odd, not to mention extremely unhealthy if you're 'happy' 24/7, 365 days a year. If you do, then you're just lying to yourself.

Saying this though, general society's everyday stresses may not necessarily be the stresses of those who have a disability. Some aspects, yes; but not all. Disability is difficult to identify with unless you have a disability of some form or have had close people in your life with a disability.

General society tends not to deal with inaccessibility, denial and ableism. Those things aren't an issue. The general public doesn't tend to feel what it's like to not have access to somewhere, to be denied something as simple and mundane as a job, because the employer was 'uncomfortable with your disability' regardless of your qualifications, and just blatant ableism with the patronisation, sympathetic looks and assumptions, trying not to get bogged down in the process. It's a very hard and unnecessary battle people with disabilities face **every single day without fail**. This is the actual issue I'm focusing on this time around. It's needed.

People generally seem to be attracted to you when you are 'bubbly' and 'fun' and doesn't have disability, as life can be hard enough as it is, so being around those who are considered to be a 'fun' person, is a very attractive prospect, (especially if that 'bubbly and fun' person doesn't have a disability, well, that's all the better), but if that 'bubbly' and 'fun' person, without a disability develops a mental health issue of some form, then you get to see people's true colours when all bets are off, when you need help. Commonly, people with disabilities don't tend to have this issue because we're isolated anyway. Allergic to any kind of human interaction it seems.

Of course, this 'fun' personality can be a mask to hide deeper issues when out in public, people often fall for the fake you, not realising that it is a mask, that you're hiding your true feelings. When it gets too much to deal with, and fragments of your struggle starts to materialise, then people are faced with this option to indeed fight with you or flee from you.

There doesn't seem to be this fight or flee option if you have a disability of some form and suffer with your mental health. You're stigmatised as it is without adding a mental health issue on top. You are automatically treated differently as it is. Confirmation of a mental health issue only drives society further away, making the feeling of isolation more intense, and therefore making mental health issues more severe. It's a never-ending cycle of distress.

Mental health is finally being recognised today as a whole – which is great – but specific factors of why a mental health issue occurs ultimately get ignored. Case in point, disability.

In my own opinion, by in large, it's society which causes mental health deterioration in relation to disability. Admittedly, not all the time, but I would say a good 95% of mental health decline is down to ableism when disability is added into that fact.

This is why I feel the need to concentrate my third book on disability and mental health deterioration. In short, it doesn't get talked about enough, but it absolutely should. As mentioned already, mental health issues are being recognised as a whole (especially in media, *ITV's Britain Get Talking* campaign to just take one example of this progression), but to truly improve public relations and perceptions, we do need to look at and more importantly, understand the different layers of mental health in relation to different subjects.

Now is the time to understand how ableism negatively impacts on mental health decline.

There shouldn't be any more hiding from it.

It's time to learn, understand, embrace and change for the better.

Behind The Smile: Silenced

Behind the smile
You hide so many emotions.
Some good, some bad
The bad sadly outweigh the good
You just learn to 'deal'.
Deal with the discrimination.
Deal with the judgement.
Deal with the perceptions.
Deal with the rejection.
Deal with the segregation.
Deal with the isolation.
Deal with the bullying.
Just 'deal'
There's nothing more that can be done.
You try to fight.
You automatically are shut down.
You're 'vulnerable'
So, you don't have a chance.

You don't have a voice.

A mind of your own

You're not given a chance.

So

What do you do?

You learn.

Learn to 'deal'

Deal with the constant ableism.

By painting on a fake smile

Carrying on the best you can

In the face of adversity

You don't see the point in fighting anymore.

So, you don't

You smile.

A fake smile.

Suppressing your feelings

To conform to social ideals

You feel defeated.

But don't show it.

You carry on.

Pretending to be happy

Trying to end the stigma

Disability and mental health can have on a person.
But all the while
You have to fight those feelings.
As
Behind the smile
Is a
Constant
Relentless
Silenced

Chapter 1
Introduction

"Our mental health is inextricably linked with our physical and emotional health, as well as the circumstances in which we live. Sadly, evidence shows some groups and communities are at greater risk of poor mental health than others. This includes disabled people and people with a learning disability." – [Lesley Griffiths, Member of the Senedd for Wrexham]

"Am I a part of society?"

This is the question that most people who have a disability of some form find themselves asking on a daily basis sadly. I, myself have personally asked this question especially since becoming an adult. Especially becoming an adult with a physical disability. The lines of communication are automatically closed I've learned over the years, once you mention disability. It's treated as a crude word, people tend to recoil in horror when the

Introduction

disability topic is mentioned, and avoid it like the plague. Why?

In all honesty, people in general are so far removed from society today, given the media and technology factor, that it would be acceptable to make the argument that absolutely everyone asks this exact question at some point in their lives, regardless of who they are, especially in adolescence. The human race have been trained. Consumption of media and social media is ultimately making us more dependent, making the ability to make informed opinions by ourselves impossible. It's quite sad really if you think about it. Earth, renowned for having intelligent life forms, are being exposed and reduced to something that shouldn't have power over us. These things were designed and created to inform us, to connect us. All I see are robots ready to believe everything they see, read and hear because this is what is trusted by society sadly.

I keep referring back to the saying in my writing that *"Rome wasn't built in a day."* I completely understand that it's not going to change overnight, that's foolish to believe, but it doesn't help matters when we claim to be something we're not. How does this make any sense? It's clear we aren't where we should be in 2024, there's still a massive stigma around certain topics deemed "too sensitive" to approach. It seems to me that we're taking 2 steps forward and 10 steps back. This just exemplifies the issue we face as a society. Why have this mentality? What is the actual point? I'd much rather society hold their hands up and admit that we aren't equality driven, but we want to **learn**. This is the key word, learn. Often equality comes down to assuming. We assume what mental health issues are, we assume what disability is, but the thing is that these topics are so complex, nobody can ever really define them, but that's okay because you aren't meant to. I'll cover a little more on this later, but it isn't up to you, 'Joe Bloggs' to describe others, only the person living with something as a mental health issue, a disability or even both can do this. Remember, you are only seeing a glimpse of the person. The person themselves are living with that glimpse constantly, more often than not,

Introduction

in a hostile environment created by a society who are so eager to label anything and anyone, that the lines between the reality and fiction become blurred. This is when the risk of mental health decline happens. We can have an exponential crisis or mental breakdown if we, (people with a disability) are constantly barraged by ableism and labelling. I know, because I did have a mental breakdown, for this exact reason.

Now, you may be thinking, *"Here she goes again, talking about her favourite subject and how perceptions need to change. I've heard it all before."* The truth is disability isn't my favourite subject to talk about. In all honesty, I'd love nothing more than to distance myself from the label. I have so many more interesting things that I'd love to share with you, but the truth of the matter is, I have been subjected to so much scrutiny over the years because of my mild Cerebral Palsy, that it eventually took a toll on my mental health. So, excuse me if I am passionate about trying to change the narrative on disability, it's only because I know full well where that narrative can lead.

Disability and mental health do need to be spoken about and spoken about until you understand what I am actually saying. There are so many areas to consider when talking about disability. I've only just scratched the surface. People have said to me that I should stop, as I've spoken about disability now, that somehow my job is over. Really? I'm doing this as much for myself as I'm doing it for you. Writing is therapeutic for me. It takes me away from the realities I face. It's a form of counselling without actually verbally communicating, which can be daunting. I'm not writing constantly. Just in my spare time. As long as I and others are forced into this box, I'm never going to stop. Yes, I'm one more voice, but it's another voice striving for change. We have no choice in the matter. There are so many areas to consider when talking about disability, this next book is yet just another area that people. I feel, don't consider, but is equally important.

There is so much backlash, so much discrimination that unfortunately happens if you have a disability. Therefore, it is a no brainer that mental health issues are related in some way. Unemployment, lack of accessibility, lack of independence, segregation, manipulation, isolation, patronisation, discrimination, etc., are often the main contributing factors to disability and this uncertainty driven mind-set. Disability can be a lonely place.   Our entire life is shaped around our disability. It should be that our disabilities are shaped around our lives, our lives are worth a trillion times more than our disabilities, but people cannot see this, or even accept it as fact. In the overall consensus of society, a person with a disability is vulnerable. It doesn't matter who we are as an actual person, and our abilities, which doesn't matter in the slightest. What does matter is how disability has been perceived over the years. Anything to challenge this perception, ultimately gets ignored. Anything to go against the grain, as a society doesn't register, doesn't compute, this is the saddest thing. Society has become brainwashed into believing in a completely outdated notion.

Yes, of course, knowledge of disability is crucially important, but that knowledge shouldn't overshadow us as a person. If you have a disability of some form, it encapsulates you, it consumes you. It labels you. You are just a statistic, part of a demographic, nothing more. As a direct result, your mental health could be put into jeopardy if you are constantly scrutinised for something you can't control.

It is said to *"never judge a book by its cover"*, but this is exactly what society does constantly. Scrutinising others, in order to make themselves feel better. We know that we're disabled, but we don't necessarily identify as such. That knowledge of disability looks completely different from society's point of view, compared to those with lived experience. It's a toxic culture that we now live in, and I will go into why this is later, but we have become a world of judges, it doesn't matter who we are, or what we do, that judgement is always there, in the background, just watching and waiting for us all to slip up in some way. Never more so than when disability of any form is thrown in the mix, but we are **all** open to ridicule. We aren't equal society wise, but we are equal criticism wise. Everyone is eligible for backlash, nobody is immune, but no-one is eligible for a standard part of life. It's a level playing field when it comes to criticism.

We should ultimately be grateful for any scrap of dignity it seems, any suggestion of independence? The number of people who sadly have experienced this is unfathomable. This is cruel, old-fashioned and just plain wrong on so many levels.

This constant *Big Brother* type of surveillance is damaging us as a human race. Every little detail of our lives is being watched in some way, and this behaviour lends itself to mental health deterioration. Sometimes severe, sometimes mild, but mental health deterioration all the same.

We are actually playing out George Orwell's book, *Nineteen-Eighty-Four*. We believe everything we read or are told by people in power, and just accept it as fact without question. We have become brainwashed. The world has become despondent to rational, independent thought. This is the frightening thing. To go from achieving in the past such as winning World War II for example, to go from that to then develop this reliance on being told what to think, is a major step backwards.

We are living in 2 different societies at exactly the same time:

Orwellian **and** Dickensian.

This will hopefully make sense as you read further.

There's a legitimate argument to be made that this privacy issue has on society today, is harming the whole of society's mental health. People generally become obsessed and addicted to this life of intrusiveness because it's so easy to execute. This is an addiction. We are fascinated by finding out more and more about something. Never more so than on social media.

We care about our online personas today and how we're perceived by others in that online world, I would argue we care more about this fake lifestyle than our actual real lives. Our physicality has become secondary to our virtual life. The reason why people are so dependent on social media – I feel – is the belief that we can control the narrative.

Introduction

We have a choice on how we're perceived, which is untrue, this is the mask. Social media puts on this persona itself that people have the power to decide, but really, it's the media world in general which ultimately has the power. That's the 1 thing that is pulling the strings. The 1 common denominator. This is horrifying that we have become so dependent on technology. In truth, technology has all of the power, and we are just the slaves to devices.

It's funny and ironic to me that we often turn to social media to create a new life for ourselves, a persona, a fantasy. There's a choice. Yet, a person with a disability doesn't have that choice of creating a new life, a new persona, as that stigma is always there, hanging over them (us), the elephant in the room. Even if we try to create a new way of life for ourselves, we're ultimately held back by the disability. Society cannot let go of the perception.

We cannot place judgement on other demographics publicly at least. That's frowned upon. However, somehow, it's okay to judge those with a disability? How is that fair? How does this make any sense at all? Think about that for a while. Let that sink in.

Being exposed to absolutely everything all at once can really have a detrimental effect on a person's mental health. Feeling overwhelmed by everything that you see and hear constantly can cause depression, anxiety, alongside a whole host of other mental health issues. Mental health issues that are caused by social media can include:

- Negative expectations

- Judgement

- Bullying

- Comparison

- Disruption of sleep

- Inappropriate content

- Lacking concentration

- Lack of privacy

- Racism

- Ableism

Introduction

-
- Homophobia
- Harassment

Alongside other serious factors.

This is why I now feel it's time to talk about mental health and its connection with disability. I've spoken about mental health in parts in both *CP Isn't Me* and *Disabling Ableism*, but I haven't yet written a book that is solely dedicated to highlighting mental health in relation to disability. My past conversations on mental health have been in a chapter format. Yes, I've touched on the subject a bit, but not as much as I would've liked. I want to delve deeper. Questions need to be asked. *Silenced* is going to open up that conversation more, by dedicating an entire book to the subject.

When we talk about disability, there are so many areas to consider. Most people focus on the disability itself without considering the person behind, or even the mental impact those disabilities and/or reactions may have on those people. There's no connection there. People with disabilities are almost always treated like objects, devoid of human emotions. Nobody actually realises or takes the time to understand that we are human first and foremost. I do get that the subject of disability can be daunting, you don't know how to approach it, so I bet your way to deal with it is to avoid and ignore us? We're monsters right?

Mental health can be considered a minefield in itself, again with so many areas to consider, but it has had a recent insurgence in people wanting to learn more about mental health as a standalone topic, and how important it actually is, alongside how we can maintain it. There's this realisation now, in part thanks to campaigns such as *ITV's Britain Get Talking*, and of course, the recent COVID-19 pandemic, where mental health was at the forefront of the world. It was a global concern, only second or third to the pandemic itself.

When it comes to disability and specifically, disability's connection to mental health, there's very little (if any) interest in the subject. I think this is because everyone has a mind, and therefore,

Introduction

everyone has mental health, but not everyone has a disability, so I feel this is why disability and mental health generally get ignored. So, *Silenced* is going to focus on the disability side of mental health and how perceptions of disability impact on a person's mental health. Of course, I will delve a little into different factors of mental health deterioration, but my main focus for this book is mental health's relationship to disability. I will look at different factors such as social/societal, environmental and personal, to see if there's any correlation.

I just want to make it clear that in no way am I downplaying the legitimate other reasons as to why mental health issues may occur, I just have a lot of personal experience with disability and mental health to draw from. Every reason is valid, I've experienced loss and hardship in my life like everyone else, which of course took a toll on me mentally, but sadly, my own disability has taken precedence with regards to my mental health journey above anything else, especially in recent years. It may seem selfish, but I'd rather write about something I know well and write in depth, than to do tons of research only to have a short piece on the subject. In this case, quantity is equal to quality. It's extremely important to highlight different areas of mental health, how different lifestyles can have a profound impact on our mental health, and disability is definitely one to give a spotlight to.

I've decided with this book to combine the format of *CP Isn't Me* and *Disabling Ableism*. I'm going to talk more about my own personal mental health journey, but I will also add research. As with *Disabling Ableism*, any quotes I use will be emboldened to differentiate between my own story and research. I have again been so lucky to have establishments and Government backing in the form of the *House of Commons*, alongside the *House of Lords* who have kindly granted me permission to quote from them as and when needed. Mental health charities such as *Mind*, and disability charities including *Scope* and *Sense*, alongside many others, of which I wholeheartedly appreciate.

I have also asked again for public participation. Each participant has been so open and honest about their own experiences of which I am truly grateful. There's no point in writing a book like this, if it isn't going to be truthful. Nothing would be gained or learned if this was the case. In order to make the experience more comfortable for participants, I explained that they can either be credited, or remain anonymous, whichever the individual prefers. As a result, you will read some experiences from those who have agreed to be credited, however you may also read the experiences of those who have asked to remain anonymous.

It's vitally important to ask those people who live with and experience disability about their own experiences of both subjects in order to give a fully rounded view. My own experiences, and statistics are good, but in order to not be biased, having others speak on this subject will ultimately give the subject some weight. Again, I wholeheartedly appreciate every single participant's contribution, without whom, this book wouldn't be possible.

Mental health issues are common, especially with a disability. We desperately need to change our attitude on both subjects. People generally need to understand the connection between disability and mental health deterioration. Our 'modern, accepting and equality driven lifestyle' is based on a lie as it currently stands. Some areas are improving, but there's still a clear division there.

Society needs to accept that people can have a disability of some form **and have the capability to develop numerous mental health issues alongside**.

A mental health issue can affect anyone, at any one time. Absolutely nobody is immune. Mental health never discriminates unfortunately. This, it seems, is the job of society, to pass judgement on really, something that doesn't impact on the general population. It's a horrible thing when you realise that mental health isn't discriminative, but society is towards anything that is a little different or considered difficult to accept or talk about openly. The ethical implications this creates is immense to say the least.

Introduction

A lot of this mentality does come from media (especially social media). Needless to say, I will be looking at this 'modern world', a world so reliant on media, it seems that we have forgotten the ability to form opinions ourselves. I will cover this matter later.

Discrimination seems to be the go-to defence mechanism for society. This mentality desperately needs to come to an end. We cannot carry on like this. We have just become a world of insecurities.

Chapter 2
What is Mental Health?

As you may already know by now, if you have read my books before this one, I like to start off by establishing more background on the subject matter itself, before anything else. This way, you, the reader, ultimately gets to understand and acknowledge the matter from the get-go.

"Mental health is a state of mental well-being that enables people to cope with the stresses of life, realize their abilities, learn well and work well, and contribute to their community. It is an integral component of health and well-being that underpins our individual and collective abilities to make decisions, build relationships and shape the world we live in. Mental health is a basic human right." – ['Components of Mental Health', WHO, (World Health Organization)]

Everyone has mental health. Maintaining our mental health is extremely important. It helps us to navigate through life, to function. Sometimes

What is Mental Health?

though, mental health can be put into jeopardy, which can cause serious mental deterioration depending on who we are. These factors can be personal, environmental, and/or social.

In an ideal world, issues with our mental health would never be a reality, but they are a thing, as life gets in the way, and life can have numerous different negatives that can put mental strain on ourselves. Stresses such as school, bullying, friendships, relationships, money worries, exam revision and results, work stresses, the everyday stresses of life. Then, there are those stresses which can hit a little bit deeper, stresses that are a bit more serious to deal with such as, abuse (both physical and mental), trauma, poverty, violence, neglect, inequality, emotional skills, substance use, genetics and environmental deprivation, racism, homophobia, and ableism. Of course, this is dependent on the person and their personality, everyone deals with stress differently, but if overexposed to any kind of stresses, whether large or small, ultimately, they will jeopardise anyone's mental health. Nobody is immune to developing potential mental health decline.

"Mental health issues can disrupt sleep schedules, affect appetite, impact energy levels and disrupt cognitive processes and planning abilities. They can also affect motivation and make an individual less likely to engage in healthy habits, make an effort to engage socially, or take care of oneself. All of these things can aggravate or worsen any pre-existing physical health problems..." – [Richard Luke, Specialist Information Officer and Cerebral Palsy Programme Lead, Scope]

Issues with mental health can materialise at any stage of life. It differs from person to person. This is subjective. Mental health issues are also subjective. People have different reactions to what they can mentally deal with. Some people react to stress instantly, and depending on the person and the situation, people can also have delayed reactions to stress which can impact negatively on our mental health down the line.

What is Mental Health?

Some things that can contribute to developing potential mental health issues are:

- Bullying

- Domestic abuse (physical and/or mental)

- Money worries

- Unemployment

- Traumatic events (military combat, being involved in a serious incident in which you feared for your life, or being the victim of a violent crime)

- Sleep deprivation

- Bereavement

- Childhood abuse, trauma, or neglect

- Poverty

- Debt

- Discrimination (racism, homophobia, ableism, etc.)

- Isolation

- Loneliness

- Long term stresses

- Life threatening situations

- Rejection

- Relationship breakdown

- Homelessness

- Diet

- Being a long-term carer for someone

- Drug and alcohol misuse

- Manipulation

- Disability

It can be absolutely anything that can trigger a mental health issue. There's no one cause. It depends on the person and the situation.

What Is Being Done to Rectify This?

"In recent times, the Welsh Government has reiterated it remains focused on reducing waiting times for mental health support and treatment.

What is Mental Health?

In the longer term, the Welsh Government's dedicated Minister for Mental Health & Wellbeing hopes to "transform services" and to strengthen the government's approach to improve mental health and well-being. The major work in this area is ongoing and earlier this year (2024), the Welsh Government consulted on two key policies – the draft Mental Health and Wellbeing Strategy, and the draft Suicide and Self-harm Prevention Strategy. The responses have provided Welsh Government with valuable information. Many are generally supportive of the cross-government approach to tackle the wider detriments of mental health but the need to provide greater "person-centred and needs-led support" is clear." – [Lesley Griffiths, Member of the Senedd for Wrexham]

As it currently stands, waiting times for mental health support in general is appalling. Knowing the Welsh Government is looking into the issue is something, however actions speak louder than words. Usual waiting times are diabolical within A&E for example, with people having to sleep on hospital floors due to lack of beds, ambulance waiting times etc., as it is. I just hope that Welsh Government come good on their promises, and fast.

Recently, as of writing this, (November 2024) the UK Government has announced a new mental health bill. It's admitted by the UK Government that mental health standards aren't where they should be, and so this new bill promises to:

- *Outdated Mental Health Act modernised to better support patients, treat them more humanely and address disparities*

- *Reforms will introduce statutory care and treatment plans, end the use of police and prison cells to place people experiencing a mental health crisis, and end the inappropriate detention of autistic people and people with learning disabilities*

- *Greater involvement of patients, families and carers will improve treatment while*

What is Mental Health?

protecting patients, staff and the wider public

[Information from UK Government – Published 6th November 2024]

Currently, people experiencing severe mental health issues are thrown in police cells, and as it currently stands, the law automatically gives the power of decision making to a nearest relative, rather than asking the person suffering a mental health issue the choice of who they would like.

This new law aims to tackle such Dickensian thinking.

Now, this is still in the early stages, but if the bill delivers on what it promises in delivering significant changes in attitudes towards mental health, then it will be a step in the right direction especially with disability because:

"Black people are over 3 times more likely to be detained under the act, while those with a learning disability and autistic people are also found to be inappropriately sectioned. Patients

currently have little say over their care and treatment should they be detained, or over who should be involved in making decisions related to their care, such as family members and carers." – ['Mental Health Act reformed to improve treatment of patients and address disparities.', Published: 6th Nov 2024, Department of Health and Social Care, NHS England, Lord Timpson OBE and The Rt Hon Wes Streeting MP, GOV.UK]

This mistreatment only encourages dependency. This new bill hopefully will rectify these issues to help society be a truly equality driven world.

Will this be enough? Can we do more? Baby steps I suppose, we must start somewhere.

"Whereas governments can focus on enhancing the availability of support, it is also vital we increase awareness, understanding and compassion within services and society generally, so people can feel confident to reach out without fear of stigma or judgement. The current situation is far from perfect and there is clearly

What is Mental Health?

still work to do, however, I do feel, in my 17 years as being the Member of the Senedd for Wrexham, that more people are recognising mental health matters." – [Lesley Griffiths, Member of the Senedd for Wrexham]

All I can say is, time will tell on all these things.

Chapter 3
Disability and Mental Health

So, that's society's, and the Government's stance on mental health, quite a confusing view in my opinion, as in a way the relationship is getting better, but not so much if 2024 is the first year by Government for potential action on delivering mental health reform.

All mental health issues are serious whether they are mild, moderate or severe, but this doesn't mean that people should be treated any differently from the next person. Same argument with disabilities. We are becoming more aware, especially with mental health, but it's a slow progression, case in point, disabilities. The fear of the unknown keep people at bay from learning and understanding. People generally like to observe from a distance, not participate in shaping a society that actually works alongside topics to make them more ingrained into the public consciousness, breaking down barriers along the way. If society's claims were

Younger Years

brought to Trading Standards somehow, then it wouldn't surprise me in the slightest to see the whole of society be reprimanded for their claims, as the reality is so different. I wish there was a system for this, but it wouldn't actually be humane, and sadly, I doubt effective as people would no doubt find loopholes in order to avoid being reprimanded. Yes, there's the police. Law enforcement is a part of society, but sometimes the law does let people down, and judgement still happens regardless of the law.

"There is no offence of stirring up hatred based on disability, which contrasts with the position in relation to offences of stirring up hatred on grounds of race, religion and sexual orientation." – ['Disability Hate Crime and other crimes against disabled people – prosecution guidance', Updated: Mar 3rd 2022, CPS.gov.uk]

This right here, is one of the reasons why people with disabilities can suffer from mental health issues. This complete disregard for disability, as if we don't matter.

Things do take time to perfect, I do appreciate this, but for the CPS (Crown Prosecution Service) to

Disability and Mental Health

blatantly admit this on their website, says a lot about the current state of affairs and how even the law views things such as disability. Disability Hate Crime is serious and can cause serious implications to a person albeit physical, mental and/or emotional. It's disgusting. This just goes to prove my point that people with disabilities are treated as second class citizens and disproportionately affected by a system Hell-bent on creating more barriers. However, it's confusing because the same website, (actually the same page on the website) goes onto list examples of Disability Hate Crime and what needs to be done whilst considering if it's an actual hate crime. Contradiction at it's finest.

I'm sorry, but anyone using ableism, ableist language, and/or tactics is hate crime in my book, (pun intended). Things are created to make a person intimidated, and not want to bother making a complaint. We shouldn't be deterring, we should be encouraging. No hate crime is superior to another. It should be equal, and information should be simple. A person with ADHD or autism wouldn't be able to cope with the amount of information on the website. It's overwhelming. I was even a bit overwhelmed with how much information was added, and I only have a mild form of Cerebral Palsy. Just imagine what it would be like in that situation, well, I say imagine, nobody can unless you actually know what it's like, and not just casually say *"I know what you're going through, I was in a wheelchair for a week once."* News flash, no you don't, you've seen a glimpse again, had a small taster. There's so much more than just sitting in a wheelchair for a week. After that week, you probably are back to how you used to be before the wheelchair. The wheelchair is just something to sit in whilst you heal, for us, it's so much more, you can't even begin to imagine. It's an object of ridicule, of humiliation, of plain ignorance to most people in society. A wheelchair is an object, so by extension, we also become part of that object. We, the living, breathing person disappears, consumed by our 'props'. We ultimately become identified as a disability. The 'disability' comes first in the description. A person with a disability is often referred to as the *"disabled person/people"*. Now,

Disability and Mental Health

this maybe okay for some with a disability, it's preferred, which is absolutely fine, it's **their choice**. Often though it doesn't become a choice, it becomes normalised, and we're are just expected to accept that? This can play a significant role in mental health deterioration. We should be **allowed** to make decisions about how we would prefer to be identified, it's a basic human right. When you have a disability however, 9 times out of 10, our basic human rights are taken away from us, simply because we're seen as that object.

If the website was purposely designed like that by the CPS and Government, not only in layout, but language, then it's shameful. I would like to believe that it's an oversight designing the website in such an overwhelming way and obviously ableist tone, but even oversights shouldn't happen today. We as a human race should have the common sense to recognise when things are wrong. We are **supposed** to be the intelligent race after all.

I wholeheartedly believe the reason why things such as race, religion and sexual orientation for example get more time and respect by the law is simply because the subjects are a part of society. Justice doesn't happen constantly with these subjects if there's a hate crime aimed towards one of these demographics, justice doesn't happen all the time, but they are more likely to obtain justice rather than a disability case, I personally feel, because people with disabilities are mistreated every single day anyway regardless, so why shculd we expect to be heard by the law? It's just a constant silence. There should never be a decision process. The information on the actual website is longwinded and daunting. The website in itself can be considered as anxiety inducing in itself, given the amount of information on the website. I do wonder if this is deliberate? Whether because people with disabilities are treated as second class citizens, if this actually is a tactic to keep Disability Hate Crime at bay, keeping up the pretence of an 'equal opportunities for all society' truly at the heart of the public consciousness, deceiving and manipulating ourselves in the process? Brainwashing in fact?

Disability and Mental Health

It's about time we look at this area of disability. An area, I feel gets overlooked quite often because disability is just seen as a disability and nothing more. We're objects, not humans. Robots in fact avoid of human emotions it seems. I want to challenge this. I want to open your eyes, open you up to the realities of disability and see if mental health issues in people with disabilities are negatively affected. Something that I feel doesn't have enough exposure, (if at all).

Is it environmental, physical, personal, social/ societal, or indeed, all of the above? As you will read a bit further on in this chapter, Richard Luke, Specialist Information Officer and Cerebral Palsy Programme Lead at *Scope*, said that certain conditions are more susceptible to mental health decline, but in contrast, untreated mental health issues can lead to potential issues with physical health. A catch 22.

Arguably, I've experienced both instances. I accept that having a condition can increase the risk of developing a mental health issue, but it's also true that mental health issues can cause physical health deterioration, but is that increase in mental health deterioration from disability, actually a personal response of a disability itself, or from outside influences such as mistreatment? There's an argument for both cases really in my own personal opinion.

"Amongst disabled working-age adults the most prevalent impairment type reported were mental health impairments, with 47% reporting this kind of impairment. The second most prevalent type of impairment were mobility impairments at 41%. For state pension age adults with a disability, the most common impairment type were mobility impairments at 69%. The second most prevalent impairment type was a stamina, breathing or fatigue impairment at 46%. Among disabled children the most common impairment type was a social or behavioural impairment at 50%." – ['Challenges faced by people with disabilities', Charley Coleman, Published: Mon, 13 May 2024, House of Lords Library]

This 1st statistic is exactly why I felt it necessary to write about disability and mental health in the 1st place, with a staggering 47% of the population of people with a disability in the UK, experiencing issues with their mental health. It just goes to prove that the mental health of a person with a disability can significantly worsen, and so is relevant. It's not just me surmising. This is a cold, hard fact from the *House of Lords*. For mental health issues to take precedence over actual mobility issues really says where we are as a society, if mobility issues are 2nd in importance of concerns. This only justifies my reasoning to write such a book.

This fact can also be backed up by the *House of Commons*:

"People living with long-term physical health conditions are two to three times more likely to experience mental health conditions than the general population. In addition, people with long-term conditions that experience mental health problems are more likely to experience poorer outcomes in their physical health and quality of life..." – ['Mental health and long-term conditions', Published: May 14th 2024, House of Commons Library]

Government is clearly aware of the issue, and this is why the new bill is so important and should be treated as such. It should be obvious to anyone that if people, especially with disabilities, are dehumanised and mistreated by being placed into police cells and having their rights taken away, then of course, the likelihood of a mental health issue developing increases. It's distressing and humiliating to say the least.

A Catch 22

"Mental and physical health are deeply interconnected. While chronic health conditions such as Cerebral Palsy (CP) can increase the risk of developing anxiety or depression, untreated anxiety or depression can also contribute to poor physical health..." – [Richard Luke, Specialist Information Officer and Cerebral Palsy Programme Lead, Scope]

When I was in the midst of my mental health decline, I developed chest pains, red bumps on my skin, blurred vision, shaking, palpitations, heartburn, migraines, and mouth ulcers. I also used

Disability and Mental Health

to suffer quite badly from panic attacks. I didn't like to be left alone for too long, otherwise I'd experience those heart palpitations, sweats, shakes, and I'd be on the phone to mum until she got back home, which is very unlike me. Usually, I love being on my own, I love my own company. If mum and dad go out in the week to run errands, I prefer to be at home. That's my time to unwind and enjoy a bit of self-care. Do what I want to do for a few hours. During the darkest period of my mental health issues, this didn't exist, I couldn't enjoy being me. I needed someone with me 24/7 to take my mind off my thoughts. It was in that silence when the noise in my mind would decide to rear its ugly head. I needed constant distraction from my own head. It wasn't a nice place to be. I had some extremely dark thoughts during this time, including self-harm and suicide sadly. I just didn't want to feel the way I was anymore in my own head.

Although during this time, I didn't really feel anything at all either. I was numb, depressed, couldn't be bothered with anything. I felt nothing, but to counteract this, I felt emotional, angry, anxious. It was like two wars were going on within me on a daily, and sometimes hourly basis, and none of them good. It was just tiring, but there was nothing I could do to stop the deterioration. Certain people in my life at this point significantly contributed to my mental health decline, coupled with the relentless mistreatment from general society on a daily basis I somehow also had to contend with. I had to contend with manipulation, gas-lighting, and empty promises from these certain people. They lived to see me suffer, and they enjoyed it. I was under their spell. I couldn't see them for what they were, because in a warped way, I became devoted to them. They knew this, and instead of stopping the mistreatment, it only increased. I became so enamoured with these people, in my eyes at the time, they could do no wrong. I do think that becoming so unsure about myself, looking for reassurance constantly, I think this only blinded me to the truth of what was actually happening. Any form of mistreatment from these people, I actually blamed myself for. Lying to my face by saying that they were away for the

Disability and Mental Health

weekend when I invited them to a concert, only to discover that they weren't away at all, it goes without saying, hurt me significantly. They don't know that I know what happened as I've already explained in CP Isn't Me, as I kept it hidden from them sadly. I just didn't want to admit to myself that I was being mistreated yet again. I pushed this, and many other instances to the back of my mind. I had to, otherwise what else would I have? I do believe it was an attempt to save any shred of self-respect I had left ironically. I kept everything quiet, but as I would soon discover, keeping everything locked up inside would only exasperate the issues, not prevent them. If I spoke up, I would only be playing into society's beliefs of disability. I didn't want to give society the ammunition to double down on the negative perceptions of disability. So, I continued to be in contact with these certain people, to save face, to give the illusion of a successful life. By deciding to eliminate these people, I would also be eliminating the chance for proper disability awareness and inclusion. Obviously, I didn't want to jeopardise this any further. So, I kept quiet for so many years whilst knowing them. I was in awe to put it mildly. I would go as far as to say that I worshipped the ground these people walked on. They were introduced in my life at an extremely fragile period of time. I didn't know what was up or down, left or right. I was confused and in desperate need of some attention. These certain people, I feel thrived on my mental pain, they must have if I was constantly experiencing mental anguish. There logically cannot be another reason, unless it was a case of misunderstanding, but the cynic in me says it can't be as it was obvious these certain people knew what they were doing and **chose** to continue. It was cruel.

No wonder I eventually had a mental breakdown as a result. I just couldn't take anymore difficulties, anymore ableism, anymore manipulation. I didn't deserve it. You work hard during your education in the belief that you will be sought after by the qualifications you have, not shunned because of your life. That's just wrong and should **never** be allowed to happen.

Disability and Mental Health

People shouldn't manipulate you because they think they can, they shouldn't give you false hope, they shouldn't lead you on, they shouldn't gaslight you, they shouldn't make empty promises, they shouldn't patronise you, they shouldn't discriminate you, they shouldn't compare you on image alone. This mistreatment would play with anyone's mind regardless of who they are. Tell me, how is this fair?

You shouldn't have to deal with such cruelty and evilness. Nobody should.

That mental breakdown was my mind giving up, after keeping up the pretence of a well-rounded individual for so long. I just couldn't pretend anymore. It was a delayed response. It was as if a knot was tightening in my mind, giving me severe headaches to the point of migraine. Nothing I did ever felt right to me, I was in a constant state of doubt, the panic and fear became too much, not for only myself, but my family too. I became my biggest critic. I think this is where I developed OCD (obsessive compulsive disorder), the doubt made me question my actions. I checked everything daily, then I rechecked everything until it felt right in my head. Nothing was ever simple. I would really be obsessed with keeping everything safe and secure. Things had to be done a certain way, otherwise I couldn't sleep. I was constantly on high alert, I didn't have a life, I just existed to check things, then recheck them. Thank God for mum during this time. I really don't know how she coped with me, because she unfortunately had to bear the brunt of my OCD. There were rules that had to be followed to the letter, otherwise, I'd make mum redo something until it was settled in my mind. I became very particular. Bless mum, because she'd understand and help me during this time. I though, was sick of how I was, who I became. I think this is why I had the breakdown. I just had enough. I couldn't take any more mental torture. I exploded.

That breakdown didn't help certain people realise their actions towards me however, it would take another good few years before I finally found the strength to let these certain people go.

It's interesting what mental health issues can do to your physical health. This is what society doesn't understand. They think a disability is just that, a

Disability and Mental Health

disability, there's no attempt to try and fully understand what disability **actually** means. The level of disrespect is palpable. It's quite understandable to come to the conclusion that people don't realise that a person with a disability can also develop physical issues as a result of mental health issues. I had to go to A&E in the early hours of the morning when my physical issues arose. When I was eventually seen, I was just told to, (and I quote), "stop worrying." As if it was that easy. A lot had happened to me up to that point in my life, close family members passing away, blatant and **continued** ableism, from being in a situation at the time where I felt disrespected and devalued. Being told to "stop worrying" as if this was a great solution to my issues, as if it was that easy, does say a lot about the relationship between society, mental health issues and disability. It just proves that people aren't educated in these important topics, and education is vital to be an actual modern world. Yes, mental health is covered more in media today, there's a surge in getting awareness of mental health out there in the public consciousness, but disability doesn't seem to have the same level (if any) of coverage, let alone linking disability to mental health. The two don't seem to connect in people's minds. Topics are separate from one another, ironically segregated in a way.

The mental health of a person with a disability often gets overlooked and overshadowed by the disability itself. It isn't just me that believes this sadly, a lot of the participants think the same. This is telling. I can imagine if you have a hidden disability of some form, it's more likely harder to be recognised for your disability and potential mental health issues.

It's also a tricky thing to navigate through if a mental health issue fluctuates, by this, I mean, one day you may feel strong enough to do something like go outside, but that doesn't mean that you necessarily will be fine going out the next day, as Rachel Williams explains:

"I think this one is harder for people to understand, as people can't see the difficulty. Like, for example, my mental health, if I can't do

something due to anxiety, I find that harder to explain to people. You have to tell them what your issue is and often they don't understand how that can affect a person. It's a lot harder to explain. When people see me, they see I can't go up a flight of stairs, but they won't see when I can't leave the house due to anxiety. Even when you explain it people usually will say things like," well you went out yesterday and you were fine?" It's hard to explain that it can be variable and can change quickly. Also, we all have the same emotions, but we experience them differently, that makes it hard for people to understand as someone might say "well I experience anxiety, and I manage to do things." Not everyone will go through the same things and experience them in the same way." – [Rachel Williams, social media participant]

It is a tricky thing to navigate, but mental health issues are often based on the assumption that everyone experiences a mental health issue in the same way. This, strangely, is the overall common belief. Everyone is individual, everyone's experience is unique, and the way we deal with situations are individual. Some people may not have any issues with different situations, and can cope with what life throws at them, but for others, this can be an extremely distinct experience, t is based on the person. Also, you may feel strong one day, but not as strong the next. It is personal. You should never be judged for how you deal with situations, you can give advice or support, but you should never manipulate people. You should not have to explain yourself either. When you have a disability of some form, you are just expected to explain yourself. The intrusiveness and blatant disregard for privacy goes out of the window. It isn't fair at all that we cannot have a sense of dignity. Dignity is a word that doesn't exist in the disability dictionary. Other people in society are accepted for who they are (for the most part) today. Why can't we have the same level of respect? Why do we have to explain when others don't? How we handle different situations is more closely monitored if you have a disability. We are put under surveillance. We are 'treated with care', just like a good tea set. We

Disability and Mental Health

are placed in metaphorical bubble wrap because we are incapable to live a relatively independent lifestyle. We cannot be trusted to do so. I have news for you though, something that I've mentioned before. Everyone deals with mental health issues differently. You should **never** influence or question people's handling of a situation regardless of who they are. It's immoral to say the least. If the choices aren't life threatening to themselves or others around them, then you have no business in trying to control a person. I do believe that it's much harder for society to accept that a person with a disability can also have a mental health issue, as it's another layer of unknown. This unknowingness can play a significant role in how society treats others as it is, nevertheless, a person with a disability.

Disability can be a daunting subject for many, even the person with a disability believe it or not. As a person with a disability myself, I came across so many barriers, that I became scared to approach people for that fear of rejection. In a way, I guess you could say, I became the stereotypical 'disabled' person. Every encounter from secondary school age onwards was extremely painful for me. Everyone had a preconceived idea of me before I even opened my mouth. People distanced themselves away, and I in turn, distanced myself away from everything and everyone, including myself. Having to fight to be recognised for **who you are instead of what you are** can be exhausting to say the least. By the end, I just gave up fighting. What was the point? It didn't matter what I did, or what I said, that preconception was always there with me, so in the end, sadly, I just decided to embrace the stereotype for years after. It was the manipulation and patronisation that really irritated me. I was treated as unintelligent, and I was disrespected constantly. It was a catch 22. I couldn't speak up for myself as society wouldn't allow it, and because I didn't speak up for myself, people treated me abominably. I couldn't win.

This is the case for so many people with disabilities.

Control

Disability and Mental Health

This is another example of disrespecting disability. Controlling behaviour. The false narrative that disability is equal to vulnerability is at the forefront of people's minds when they decide to control a person with a disability. Initially, this control may come from a place of innocence, wanting to help a person with a disability make 'better choices', but by doing so, is only discouraging the person's sense of independence and decision making. A person with a disability may become more reliant on the controlling person, because simply, they don't trust their own judgement to make decisions independently. There may be that sense of doubt and so, by letting a controlling person actually control you, you are actually giving them even more control over you, and the person may begin to feel a sense of power and confidence to take the controlling behaviour a little further, heading into coercive control territory. These scenarios are hypothetical yes, but legitimate scenarios all the same.

Personally, I've experienced this level of disrespect during certain times of my life. Controlling me because some people thought they could. Giving certain people a God complex as a result, which in turn, only increased the control that I was facing. People thought they could control me because they thought I was vulnerable, and so, took full advantage of the situation. It was an endless cycle. At certain points in my life, I was considered vulnerable. I admit I was, but vulnerable in the sense of a response to the blatant ableism I faced on a daily basis. Not vulnerable because of my mild Cerebral Palsy. This is the difference that deserves to be recognised by the public. The irony is I became vulnerable from people's perceptions of my disability, not the disability itself. I just find this interesting.

Hero Complex – Switching the Blame

People find it difficult to blame themselves, (which is a great psychological analysis, and interesting to look at in more detail), but I'm not going to research this in this particular book, as it would take the subject matter in a completely different direction.

Disability and Mental Health

Blame is generally placed on disability. A person with a disability cannot do this or that without assistance. What I will say here is that because disability is seen as a vulnerability, people in general society can (and often do in my experience) find it easier to gas-light a person with a disability, simply because they believe that having a disability is somehow weaker. Can I ask you, what about those individuals who develop a disability of some kind in later life? Are these people suddenly vulnerable? How does this make sense? Would you suddenly treat a person as vulnerable just because they've developed a disability? Would you suddenly consider yourself as superior? Disabilities from birth or disabilities in later life shouldn't have any bearing on us as individuals.

You see, non-disabled people in society are often painted as superior, they are the heroes ready to save the helpless disabled person. It's the role the non-disabled person was born to play. It's something that isn't based in reality, it's just what society has been told over the years. This is known as Hero Syndrome. It's this self-assurance that can have a significant negative impact on a person, and by extension, others around them.

How many of you have come across a person with a disability and offered assistance? You may think that you are being kind, but has the person actually **asked** for assistance or have you assumed based on appearance alone?

We are crossing into ableism here, but because of the assumption, you may make a person with a disability feel inferior in comparison. It's a careful line we have to cautiously tread admittedly, you may not know what to do next time, but I'll tell you, start a conversation before asking if the person needs help. Yes, it's simple, but effective. Create a scenario where the person doesn't feel different from the outset. Wait until they ask you. Don't take away dignity. This hero complex needs to be eradicated, and this is the best way to do exactly that. It creates equality by opening up a dialogue 1st, eliminating potential ableism in the long run. We just want and deserve to be treated as who we are, human beings first and foremost.

Disability and Mental Health

'Facts'

Quite recently, as of writing this, I had a social worker visit me at home to apparently "catch up on things". The person was lovely, don't get me wrong, they are massive believers of disability equality, but there again, this social worker was still training by going to university, studying whilst doing practical work out in the community. My mum and I could tell that this trainee social worker obtained their information from textbooks, as what they were saying was a generalised overview of my Cerebral Palsy. There wasn't any personalisation there at all. I completely understand that training is vital for jobs such as social work. It's crucial in fact. I just wish that a bit more individuality would materialise. It's okay reading 'facts' from a document, but those 'facts' never tell the story of an individual. 'Facts' aren't personal, lived experience is. You can have all the 'facts' you want, but at the end of the day, it's the person that matters. 'Facts' are generic, they are just a generalised overview of a disability. All disabilities are different. It's individual based. Nobody is going to have every single 'fact' as part of their disability. That's impossible. People may have a few symptoms on a sheet, but not everything. It's vitally important to understand this. By reeling off 'facts', you are taking away our personalities, our individuality. It makes us feel insecure, insignificant and a statistic, not a human being. Our self-esteem is put into jeopardy.

Different Fears

Can I ask you; you sometimes don't feel like getting up to go to work, there's that dread that sets in sometimes, am I right? Well, it's exactly the same in a way, if not worse for a person with a disability and mental health issues. These issues are legitimate and should never be taken lightly. The difference is that you may only have fears about work, money, bills etc., arguably the mundane lifestyle of the world. A person with a disability can develop fears of being judged, patronised, bullied, segregated, scrutinised, unemployed etc., on a daily basis for wanting to be a part of that mundane lifestyle.

Disability and Mental Health

Rachel's point of it's harder to explain a mental health issue rather than a physical disability confirms my own belief. It is much harder to explain a mental health issue rather than it is to explain a physical disability. A physical disability is obvious, mental health issues, not so much. I of course, can attest to this. The physical is more accepted in a way than the psychological. People generally can register in their minds if it is physical, in plain sight for all to see. They can identify the physical, (but that registration doesn't mean that the identification is correct, as already established), but people can pick out a physical disability, rather than a mental health issue, because simply, a physical disability is visible. However, none should take precedence. Disability and mental health should have respect, and the same level of respect for that matter. Mental health issues aren't always visible, so can fall under the radar with a lot of society. Some people with mental health issues can also develop physical signs (issues) of their struggle which can affect their physical health, only then, is there a chance of getting proper help and support, but not everyone. It is that main character syndrome which I touched upon in *Disabling Ableism* why I feel that this is true. People are the main character in their own lives, yes, we may interact and love one another, but at the end of the day, we are our only focus.

"...Ignorance is bliss..." – ['Ode on a Distant Prospect of Eton College', Poem written: 1742, Thomas Gray]

If it doesn't affect/benefit us, then generally, we pay no mind to it. This definitely can be the case for the disability and mental health topics. This ignorance mentality though, can have profound negative effects on society's understanding.

Mantras of Intrusion

Having to explain everything constantly can be draining on both the physical and the mental side of things whether you have a disability of some form or not. One's mental health issue shouldn't have to be put on display if you choose not to. It's private at the end of the day. It should be left up to the individual whether they want to divulge such

Disability and Mental Health

personal information, however, you may feel like you have to in order to be recognised. Admitting such things can be humiliating. People tend (or choose not to) make any attempt to understand, which is the most heart-breaking thing. We are known in British culture to have this 'Stiff Upper Lip' mentality to the rest of the world. Arguably, this is what Britain is famous for, having a choice to be able to keep quiet if we so choose. It comes from World War II, but it has somehow stuck with us.

Unfortunately, though, this phrase doesn't extend to the disability community in 2024, as of writing this. We don't have the choice. We're forced to live this life, play this part. Disability is destined to conform to British culture by practicing said mantras including *'Keep Calm and Carry On'*. It's expected. This is what I mean when I say that we're just expected to shut up and put up. It's extremely ironic to me that mental health in general is getting more acknowledgement, and the British mantras are becoming less relevant as a result, but when mental health issues are related to disability and disability in general, this acknowledgement is non-existent. There's this disconnect that happens so regularly that it has just become a part of the British culture itself. The culture of the world in fact. It isn't questioned, because it's hidden, but hidden in plain sight. We aren't allowed to live as others in society. It isn't the done thing. Do you know how debilitating this is? To be rejected every single day of your life over something you cannot control? Punished in a way? I would love for general society to have a taster of what a person with a disability goes through every day, just to see how they would cope. That would be a very interesting experiment indeed.

In my experience, people tend to get so hung up over the disability, so much so that they forget about the person behind and their feelings. Labels and terms are used to define us. We should never have a label or term define us; we should be able to define ourselves as individuals. I personally never meet someone and say, *"Hi! I'm disabled!"* It sounds stupid right? When I meet someone, I say *"Hi! I'm Sam!"*, just like every other person in society does when they introduce themselves to another person. I give my name, not my condition. Shocking. If a person does want to know about my mild Cerebral Palsy, I'll tell them, I have no issues with this. I prefer it. You teach people by doing this. We are human beings, not an object to be scrutinised. We shouldn't be grateful for being mistreated and misunderstood. That's just cruel.

"Disabled people are more likely than non-disabled people to have mental health issues. This includes people with physical disabilities and developmental disabilities like autism. Both biological and environmental factors affect our mental health including genes, diet and life experiences. For disabled people, these factors can be heightened. People with disabilities are disproportionately affected by isolation and loneliness, both of which impact mental health. This has been made worse by the pandemic, with almost two thirds of disabled people saying they are chronically lonely." – ['Disabled people and mental health', Sense.org.uk]

Sense does speak the truth here, as a lot of the participants of this book do agree, including Rachel

Williams, who has Sacral Agenesis, (Caudal Regression Syndrome) and Spina Bifida.

Sacral Agenesis (Caudal Regression Syndrome) – Definition

"Caudal regression syndrome is a broad term for a rare complex disorder characterized by abnormal development of the lower (caudal) end of the spine." – ['Caudal Regression Syndrome', NORD (National Organization for Rare Disabilities)]

Spina Bifida – Definition

"Spina bifida is when a baby's spine and spinal cord does not develop properly in the womb, causing a gap in the spine." – ['Overview: Spina Bifida', NHS.uk]

Of course, biological factors can play a significant part in the deterioration of mental health of a person with a disability. Not being able to do everything that a non-disabled person can, can be extremely damaging to mental health, as the dangerous comparison factor can immediately

Disability and Mental Health

come into play. However, I do feel that it's vitally important to realise that environmental factors such as assumptions and patronisation affect a person's mental health when disability is thrown in the mix. I feel that environmental factors never get the same level of attention as biological factors.

How Beliefs Are Damaging to Disability

You shouldn't believe all you read or hear. This belief has played into everyday life. We are seen as vulnerable as I've mentioned before, especially in education. We are treated differently in school to the other non-disabled pupils. We are treated with kid gloves, and this treatment can lead to bullying, especially in secondary schools, which obviously can lead to mental health decline. If you are constantly treated differently to others, especially as a teenager, there's a higher risk of developing a mental health issue of some form, which can lead to further mental anguish down the road.

This is confirmed in the next quote. This is part of Rachel Williams' experience with mental health issues, in reference to her disability:

"When I was a teenager, it [disability] affected my self-esteem hugely. As an adult it has also caused anxiety, depression, post-natal depression and I also have C-PTSD which in part is the medical trauma that I have experienced due to my disability. Looking at my mental health issues, I would say though that it was actually society's perception of disability and ableism that caused these issues... My post-natal depression was triggered by ableist attitudes towards me having a baby." – [Rachel Williams, social media participant]

C-PTSD is Complex PTSD just to put it into context.

Unfortunately, Rachel's experience isn't an isolated case. Society does feel the need to interject in other people's lives, especially those who have a disability of some form. It's almost as if society feels it's their duty to intervene in other people's lives for some reason. Personally, I find it disgusting that Rachel's post-natal depression was ultimately triggered by ableist attitudes she faced just for having a baby. This is a standard part of life that any woman, (if capable) should be allowed to experience regardless of disability or otherwise. There should never be a question. It's entirely the woman's choice. A disability doesn't always mean inability like I've said before.

I understand the concerns of managing one's own health if they have a disability of some form on top of parenting a baby, but really, if the woman wants a baby, and is independent, and strong willed, having a wonderful support system around her, then there's absolutely no justification to have concerns in all honesty. It's not up to you to play God, deciding who has a baby and who doesn't, that's immoral, ableist and can trigger a whole host of different mental health issues.

"Women with disabilities feel the desire for motherhood as much as women without special clinical needs. Their fertility is often not impacted by disability and they can have children. However, several issues must be considered, depending on the physical, mental or developmental disability..." – ['Pregnancy in women with physical and intellectual disability:

psychiatric implications', National Library of Medicine]

I've said it before, and I'll say it again, your disability should never have a bearing on who you are as a person. Period. It's unfair that things such as post-natal depression can be triggered by someone who is uneducated in the topic of disability. It's not society's decision. It's the individual's decision at the end of the day. Yes there can be risks, and these risks can be associated with a disability, but there are risks with all pregnancies. This is why all potential risks can be talked through beforehand with your GP.

A disability should never be one factor to go against having a baby. To reiterate the *National Library of Medicine*, women with disabilities have the desire to have children just like every other woman who wants to experience motherhood. I just wanted to hammer it home. To counteract this, women with disabilities should have the choice not to have children if they so wish, just like every other woman who doesn't feel motherhood is for them. It's important to establish that if a woman with a

Disability and Mental Health

disability chooses not to have children, it's her choice, and not based on her disability. Yes, there can be times when a disability impacts on the ability to have children, but this is rare. Assuming a woman cannot have children because of her disability and/or the physical and mental implications this can hypothetically cause is ableist.

Personally, at this current period in time, having children doesn't appeal to me, I have Rosie and Tommy, who are lovely, and I love them dearly, but having children of my own, I'm just not there. I have a lot going on currently, so starting a relationship and having children isn't feasible for me at this current point in my life. I'm not saying never though, if the circumstances were right in the future, then why not? I'm relatively independent and healthy with a good support system around me. I'm only 32 as of writing this, so I have a few more years to contemplate this if I so choose. Knowing I have a choice to have children in the future like every other woman who can have children gives me a sense of comfort. You should never be scrutinised for wanting to have children if you have a disability, and you should never be judged for not having a child because of an unfounded belief that it's the disability preventing a woman from conceiving. A woman simply may not want to have a baby because they don't want to, it doesn't necessarily mean that they're unable to. This is a perfect example of my argument of disability is always looked upon as a negative. When disability is at the centre of the conversation, it's almost always based on what we can't do rather than what we can. It's a pessimistic outlook which can cause barriers between disability and general society. Barriers which can cause severe mental health implications if constantly exposed to, (which, let's be real, a person with a disability comes up against prejudice on a daily basis), developing a mental health issue is sadly a given. This attitude is wrong on so many levels.

Internalised Ableism

In my own personal opinion, issues with our disabilities form from a young age, and depending on your circumstances, again, in my own personal opinion, these issues arise as soon as we reach the

Disability and Mental Health

age of a teenager. I will speak more on my own personal experiences later, but it does say a lot that it wasn't just me who experienced ableism as a teenager. Nobody seems to understand how their words and actions can have dire consequences on a person. A comment or action which you may consider insignificant, can have potential detrimental effects on others. You can have more influence than you may think.

However, internalised ableism can occur even earlier in life, from birth in fact. It's the comparison factor. This is a dangerous game. Social media has had a hand in internalised ableism over the years, yes internalised ableism has been around well before the introduction of social media with media itself, but I feel social media has only exacerbated the issue to higher levels. We have been exposed to so much airbrushing on social media, alongside seeing others have 'fun' with what people post daily. What people often tend to forget or not realise is that you are only seeing a filtered version of reality. The best bits. Just because a person posts something that looks interesting and fun, it doesn't necessarily mean that their life is constantly like this. Nobody's life is. I can imagine it would be exhausting if anyone's life was busy 24/7, but because nobody puts on how boring their lives are, due to the constant threat of peer pressure I think, others can fall into the trap and begin to hate themselves for who they are, comparing. This is when dire consequences can occur.

The Teenage Minefield

Being a teenager is a minefield, especially today, but really, it is just as tough, if not more for teenagers with disabilities. Children can be cruel, but I do feel this cruelty is learned behaviour from the adults in their lives. As Janet Jackson sang in *'Living in A World (They Didn't Make):*

"Children are called the future / of an active world / they are born with spirits so innocent / 'til we teach them how to hate..." – ['Living in A World (They Didn't Make)', Janet Jackson's Rhythm Nation 1814]

This is true especially in today's world, we are innocent at birth, but we do become corrupted in a

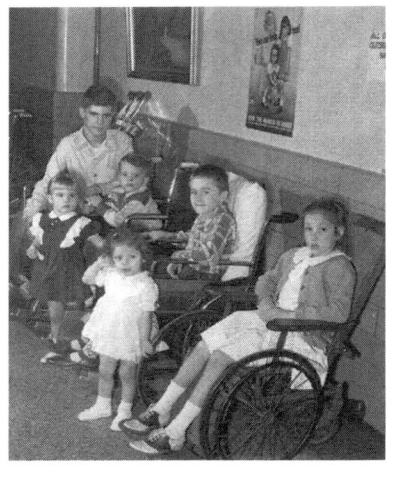

sense as we grow, gaining influence from outside sources. Children are susceptible to this, especially as they rely on adults to teach them right from wrong, but this reliance can lend itself to questionable beliefs. This of course, is dependent on the source of teachings. I think I mentioned this before, but children are like sponges, they soak up everything around them. They mimic adults both in a physical way, but also mentally in order to appear more adult themselves. This can be dangerous if the influences are irresponsible, unpopular or controversial. Adults have a responsibility to teach children. Most of the time, parents get this right, but sometimes, adults can have a negative effect on children's beliefs.

Past Mistreatment

Disability and Mental Health

The past is the past, except when it affects our beliefs in the present. Disability is such an instance. I would argue that people's perceptions of disability in the past, has greatly influenced people's beliefs today. Again, all you have to do is look at the bill that is now being reformed. Places such as asylums (left) and people such as PT Barnum have helped to perpetuate the narrative of disability is equal to difference. Exploitation and mistreatment have all helped to boost the false belief. People with disabilities being **sold** for financial gain, making ridiculous claims that people with disabilities held powers and were older than they were, in order to make a quick buck is devastating.

This negative take has trickled through to the present. Yes, it may not be as visibly ableist, but there again, today, the ableism is hidden away, which I feel is worse in many ways. Ableism isn't as noticeable today, it's covered over. Arguably, it wasn't as noticeable in the past either as there was a general misunderstanding of the subject, and the world wasn't as politically correct as it is today. It's just how the world worked back then. The political

Disability and Mental Health

correctness doesn't extend to disability today, however. We've learnt to accept certain things that we wouldn't dream of accepting years ago. We have become much more aware of our surroundings with certain topics and striving for change in certain areas, but there seems to be a reluctance to accept disabilities for some reason. This makes people with disabilities feel uncomfortable and unimportant compared to race and sexual orientation for example. We're insignificant in comparison. Unless you are willing to adapt your way of thinking fully, not just pick and choose what areas to adapt to, but actively looking to adapt in all areas, then there's absolutely no justification to adapt to other issues. It's redundant, not to mention damaging to mental health.

We were dehumanized in the past, hidden away from general society, given shock therapy or being sold as circus performers. These were the only choices a person with a disability had in the past. You can read *Disabling Ableism* to read more on this. Sadly, this hasn't improved in the slightest. We may not be as blatantly and cruelly mistreated today and exploitation may not have as much appeal as it once did, but I can argue that there still seems to be a different kind of mistreatment today, but one that is equally as bad, if not worse. As with the past, we are categorised, we're controlled, decisions are automatically made for us. We don't have a say, because we are seen as a vulnerable and incapable collective. We are not equal by any means. All this with the added pressures to look a certain way thanks to media, especially online today. Obsession, paranoia, and just general self-loathing have all helped to continue with the mistreatment of the past, morphing into something far worse. All of this mistreatment only exasperates our mental anguish. Isn't it about time that this false belief of vulnerability needs, and deserves to end? This cannot continue by any stretch of the imagination. It feels to me that general society think we're disposable. We cannot contribute to life because simply, we can't. We can't, because we're constantly being silenced. This is the truth of the matter, and God knows we deserve opportunities, equality and respect. Something that sadly,

Disability and Mental Health

disability doesn't get a lot of (if at all). I can forgive the past, because it is the past at the end of the day, there wasn't any awareness of disability inclusion, and how this mistreatment could negatively impact on a person's mental health, but there shouldn't be any excuses for blatant ableism today. Claiming to be something we are not abhorrent. We should be more knowledgeable about the subject of disability, we should be, but unfortunately, we aren't, and this is the problem.

There are still instances today where people with learning disabilities are abused by staff members whilst being housed in **specialist** mental health facilities. There are countless stories on the news to attest to this.

"The CQC re-inspected...a 41-bed inpatient facility for adults with learning disabilities and autism, in May and June after giving it a rating of "inadequate" in March... The latest inspections found that failings had not been addressed by its provider... and people continued to receive unsafe care and were sometimes subjected to abuse...CQC inspectors

also found the service did not have enough nursing and medical staff who knew the patients and was instead reliant on agency workers." – ['People with learning disabilities 'failed again' as CQC closes unit over abuse', Tom de Castella, Nursing Times, Published: 11 Aug 2021]

This is just one example of countless examples. Yes, it's no secret that the NHS is overstretched, understaffed, and as a result, stressed, the resources aren't there to cope with the ever-increasing number of patients, but this shouldn't be an excuse for abuse. There shouldn't be any excuse for abuse. It's wrong full stop. People regardless of who they are should be respected. All people should. I can imagine how frightening it must be for a person with a learning disability living in a place unfamiliar to them. Just because someone has a learning disability, it doesn't mean that people can mistreat them. I studied ethics in university, and I can tell you that this is definitely unethical. I get it, stress is running high, and nurses and staff may become frustrated, but taking this frustration out on a person with a learning disability, someone who cannot defend themselves? How have we got to this point?

Are You My Support Worker, My Carer, or My 'Handler'?

Recently, my publisher Allan and I had the opportunity to deliver talks, (which will be covered in more detail later). During the Q&A session following the speech, we were told that a certain zoo still uses the outdated and offensive term 'handlers' to describe carers and support workers. I have emailed this certain zoo to highlight the issue. It may just be a word to you, but this again can cause further barriers between disability and general society, which in turn can again cause mental health deterioration. Unless you have lived with negative terms and perceptions daily, you cannot begin to imagine the turmoil this can bring. Some terms for disability have been thankfully eradicated from society. Terms such as 'invalid' for example, alongside others have disappeared from the English vocabulary. Also, why can't a person with a disability and a non-disabled person just be friends? Why do people assume that a non-disabled person is 'looking after' the person who has a disability? It's because ableism isn't as called out as other subjects considered more important. Again, there's this unspoken hierarchy that society has created over the decades. The terms 'support worker' and 'carer' are bad enough as they only add to the negative perceptions that disability can bring. The term 'handler' only exasperates the negative perceptions and creates more of a division between disability and general society.

COVID-19 Pandemic

There was one recent significant life event which really amplified these feelings of isolation, loneliness, and fear for everyone in society, but especially for those with disabilities and the elderly population. The COVID-19 pandemic.

At its height, the recent pandemic played a significant part in the deterioration of mental health as a whole. For those with a disability and the elderly however, the impact on mental health was significantly worse. Loneliness and isolation became more apparent. Arguably, we are often

Disability and Mental Health

isolated from the rest of society anyway, but when the pandemic happened, as with everyone else, we were locked away and almost forgotten about in the grand scheme of things. It just hit home a bit more. People with disabilities, alongside the elderly may not have anyone in their lives to interact with in usual circumstances, but the pandemic, I personally feel, amplified the isolation and chronic loneliness a person with a disability and the elderly can face.

People with disabilities were labelled as more vulnerable during the pandemic, and rightly so in one regard, as people with disabilities were more likely to contract COVID-19 and depending on the individual's disability and/or condition, contracting the virus could potentially be life-threatening. This though did nothing to rectify the misconception of disability, it only cemented the stereotype in the eyes of society. Just because we were more vulnerable to the pandemic, (**to the virus**), it doesn't mean that we were actually vulnerable as a person. I think this is where the confusion comes.

The Identification Issue

Disability and Mental Health

Being identified as disabled arguably is an unfortunate thing, by social standards anyway. Once this word is placed on you, you really have no chance of a life like others, unless you are willing to fight for it constantly. You really don't have a choice.

Some challenges people with disabilities have to face are:

- Ableism
- Patronisation
- Isolation
- Loneliness
- Manipulation
- Labelling
- Vulnerability
- Unemployment
- Stigmatisation
- Dehumanisation

Disability and Mental Health

- Objectified

- Inaccessibility

- Segregation

- Judgement

- Assumptions

Alongside many other factors. These challenges are relentless. People with disabilities have to contend with this every single day. There's no break, no escape. If you're met with these challenges on a daily basis, then of course it's more likely that your mental health will deteriorate.

"On 16 May 2024, the House of Lords is scheduled to debate the following motion: Baroness Hughes of Stretford (Labour) to move that this House takes note of the challenges faced by those with disabilities including access to benefits, work, education, housing and healthcare." – ['Challenges faced by people with disabilities', Charley Coleman, Published: Mon, 13 May 2024, House of Lords Library]

Disability and Mental Health

Sense conducted a survey in 2023 asking those with severe or complex disabilities about their health and well-being.

According to *Sense*:

- **People with complex disabilities are four times as likely to say their general health is bad or very bad (25%) compared to the general public (5% according to the 2021 general census).**

- **On average, people with complex disabilities have lower happiness levels (6.02) compared to non-disabled people (7.45), according to figures from the Office for National Statistics).**

- **Those with complex disabilities have higher average rates of anxiety (5.09) compared to non-disabled people (3.12).**

- **30% of people in the UK live with one or more long-term physical health conditions, over 26% of which also have a mental health problem.**

Disability and Mental Health

- *70% of disabled people say that social isolation affects their mental health and wellbeing.*

[Information from: 'Disability and mental health statistics', Sense.org.uk]

These results are alarming but are unfortunately fact. It's well documented by now that my own mental health deteriorated significantly due to social perceptions. I worked hard throughout my educational life, overcoming hidden barriers starting from secondary school, only to be met with further rejection and manipulation at every turn. When you're considered disabled, you are also automatically considered unintelligent and vulnerable. The basis for this conclusion is unfounded and unfair. I, myself have come up against some vile mistreatment, because of this notion. It's almost as if the label gives society permission to mistreat without consequence. It's abhorrent to say the least. People often misinterpret that a disability of any kind equals a complex disability. I think that this could be the reason why those actually with complex disabilities are more likely statistically to suffer from mental health issues, as this is the overall accepted social consensus, if this makes sense? Imagine being constantly judged by strangers, people who don't know you as a **person**, yet just because you're seen as 'different' over something that you cannot control, that small insignificant 'difference' becomes your identity?

Mental health issues are often described as either a black dog, or a dark cloud. For me, it was as if a demon came into my life, telling me everything that the bullies told me in secondary school. I know that this sounds dramatic when taken out of context, but believe me, if you actually saw how I was at a particular point in my life, I can guarantee you that you would think that I was possessed. Everything just crashed on top of me one day, out of nowhere, (or so I thought). I bottled everything up for years, until my brain literally just broke down. I broke down. My mind had just had enough of the torment. Nothing actually triggered the event, it just happened. If you mistreat people long enough, regardless of who they are, that mistreatment will

Disability and Mental Health

eventually have dire consequences, not only for you, but the people around you unfortunately, which can take a toll on the mental health of those around you also. By mistreating one, you are actually affecting others who are connected to that person. It unfortunately happens, as my own family sadly can attest to. Be mindful is all I'm saying here. You do not know what your actions may cause to others.

Society has more influence than maybe first thought. Words and actions can have dire consequences. This is what society needs to understand. Of course, there's an argument to be had that society is aware of this and actively chooses to play into the ableism which is a step too far. I can unfortunately confirm that there are those who know what they're doing, and just continue anyway without a conscience. This of course will have detrimental effects on mental health, especially if you're in a position where you are unable to escape this type of abuse.

Unfortunately, the connection between disability and mental health issues are linked. I feel that society either doesn't understand the connection or, more frustratingly, ignores the fact. This conversation is important and needs to happen. It needs to be called out. Other participants think the exact same thing too.

"I don't think people understand disability. They think all wheelchair users are unable to walk when some of us can walk short distances. This impacts me mentally because I worry, I will get harassed for using the disabled parking for not being "disabled enough". "– [Rebekah Sims, social media participant]

"As a whole no. Because my disability is very visible there is more understanding but for others whose disability is less visible it is harder. It hasn't really impacted me mentally, but I am very aware of others who feel like they are being looked at as though they shouldn't be using a disabled parking space or should be contributing to society." – [Ian Jarvis, social media participant]

Two different people, who have identical feelings. One affecting their own mental health, and the other concerned for others who are worried for those who are 'unqualified' to be disabled. Both are concerning those with hidden disabilities. There are concerns by those with hidden disabilities or those who can walk short journeys but require a wheelchair for long distances.

This is a whole other issue that affects people with disabilities. Where people with physical disabilities have a battle trying to distance themselves from the label, people with hidden disabilities have a battle trying to convince society they are disabled. This just goes to show how society perceives disabilities, if we don't have a prop (wheelchair, cane, etc.,) we don't deserve the label. This can be very frustrating and degrading on both sides. What gives society the right to be judge, jury and executioner? When you either stigmatise or question a person with a disability, the mental anguish this can cause is serious.

The Questionable Questionnaires

When the then UK Government proceeded to roll out those ridiculous questionnaires which were designed to stop those in society from taking advantage by applying for benefits and other entitlements, but only served to belittle and humiliate those with disabilities, by making sure they met the 'criteria' of disability. What is the 'criteria'? What does that mean? It was horrendous in its execution. I myself had to partake in these redundant questionnaires, and I can say for certain that this wasn't well thought out. It only made people with disabilities feel more targeted by asking intrusive questions that had no relevance. A lot of mistakes were made as a result. People with disabilities paid the price. It was more like we were being judged, and judged by someone who didn't know us and our disabilities. It became apparent from the questionnaires that the UK Government designed the questions around the fictionalised version of disability, not the reality. We needed to be helpless and dependant. The only way, (it seemed at the time), was to just play up to the idea of disability. We needed to be 'vulnerable' in order to pass. It was degrading, humiliating, depressing, isolating. Some of the questions were personal,

Disability and Mental Health

some questions were downright ignorant towards disability and the person. It was clear, (to me at least), that the UK Government were out of touch with disabilities, how disability actually works and impacts us not only physically, but also mentally too. The repercussions of the experience were immense to say the least.

"How Old Are You? 18? No Social Support for You!"

It's no secret that once a person with a disability turns 18, the care from local Governments is much harder to come by. Children with disabilities are supported, but once you reach the age of 18, then really, you are lost in the system for eternity it seems.

I mean, when I was a child, my family didn't know that I was entitled to things, and (something that they wouldn't mind me saying) has had to personally pay out for things which the local Government should have been doing. Knowing what I know now, I get truly frustrated. My family has had to fight for everything for me, just for me to be able to live a comfortable, relatively independent lifestyle. I think I mentioned this before, but my mum even had to fight for some specialised scissors I was using in art class in my special education school when I was about 5 but was denied by the local Government due to budget cuts! The school I attended at the time, personally gave me a set of the scissors from their stock room after mum said we had been denied a pair of scissors. I'm a creative person, and so I personally loved art, music and creative writing from a really early age. Being denied a pair of specialist scissors which back then, probably cost a small amount was disgraceful. I was upset that I couldn't carry on my artistic skills at home, enhancing them. Creativeness was even denied to children with a disability of some form. How segregated is that? It was cruel. I can imagine the embarrassment my mum felt when she had to explain that story. I know that it was only a pair of scissors at the end of the day, but schools have budgets too. They cannot afford to be giving away equipment needed for children to learn. Especially

Disability and Mental Health

specialised equipment. It's barbaric. Those small pair of scissors caused more harm to all parties involved. Something that frustratingly, could've been avoided, just by local authorities providing one small pair of scissors.

Personal Factors of Mental Health Decline Due to Disability Issues

The human mind is a delicate, but also a complex thing. Anything can trigger a mental health issue. This obviously depends on your personal life and the situation you find yourself in.

Having a disability of some form can uncover a whole host of different factors that can contribute to developing potential mental health issues. I am going to list a few factors within this chapter, to try and educate you on how disability impacts on mental health.

It may seem unnecessary, but believe me, it definitely is necessary, as people in society have a problem with connecting the two topics somehow, (from my own personal experiences at least).

These factors may seem obvious written down, but unless I actually spell each factor out on paper, then these factors probably won't be taken seriously, and this cycle of ignorance will unfortunately continue.

Struggling To Accept Disability

The Person with A Disability

Some people find it difficult to cope with their disability. This is more suited for those who become disabled in later life, but I can imagine that there are those who struggle to come to terms with their disability from the get-go. Their mental state may not be the best from the beginning of life. Jealousy and feelings of worthlessness are factors that can develop. Seeing others live a life of ease, when you are 'limited' by yourself, can lend itself for the 'green-eyed monster' to rear its ugly head.

Now, I'm not going to divulge my opinion here, but when people are struggling to accept their disability, having the option to end your life because of it, sadly may be an attractive prospect.

Disability and Mental Health

Hidden Disabilities: Am I Disabled Enough? The Most Damaging Question and The Misrepresentation That Accelerates This Thought

There's also this stigmatisation of invisible disabilities, and the fear of not being disabled enough.

I cannot speak for those who have invisible disabilities, but I can imagine the frustration, combined with the fear of constantly being scrutinised, for not conforming to what is globally understood, (and accepted) to be disabled. The mental anguish this may cause must be significant. You can compare the attitude of invisible disabilities to mental health. The two are basically treated the same way. If it isn't physical, it doesn't matter. I've said before, but this negative attitude must be difficult to deal with daily, whether you're dealing with invisible disability backlash, or mental health deterioration backlash, it's unimaginable. To be dealing with both an invisible disability and mental health issues, well, this must be impossible. It's difficult enough when you have a physical disability, trying to be seen as more than your disability. A person who has an invisible disability arguably has the opposite fight, a fight to be recognised as a person with a disability, always being judged for not having a physical prop to 'confirm' the fact.

There's a common occurrence with society, a certain phrase, where it is thought that 'complimenting' a person, by saying that they "don't look disabled" is a good thing. Whereas, in actuality, saying this is offensive to all people with disabilities. What is a disability supposed to look like? Is there a standard that must be reached before you are labelled? Why should there always be a prop, (a wheelchair, a cane, etc.), present before a disability is accepted? A disability shouldn't have to be proven. We live in a cynical world where nothing we see or hear is accepted without proof. Always judging someone's abilities will ultimately have detrimental effects on that person's mental health if exposed to it constantly. This is what people who question, or indeed, 'compliment' those, desperately need to understand. The seriousness, and potential risk of mental anguish due to society's negative actions.

Disability and Mental Health

For example, how many of you have questioned someone who has parked in a disabled parking bay, but because they don't 'look disabled', they are automatically judged and scrutinised? Or someone who have used a public disabled facility who doesn't have something like a wheelchair or a cane to confirm that fact either.

A Global Societal Disability Fear?

There's the argument that society is fearful of disability. Fear can limit our understanding; it can limit our progression. I do wonder if this is why there's so much hidden ableism. It certainly can be considered a contributing factor.

Fear can also cause mental health issues. The anxiety and stress this fear can cause to society can be immense. People in general society can be reluctant of approaching a person with a disability because of:

- Fear of the unknown

- Lack of exposure to disability

- Fear of offending

112

- Preconceptions

- Fear of disability (ableism / anapirophobia)

- Outdated beliefs

- Misunderstanding

All these things can play a significant part in the mistreatment of disability, and these factors mostly are socially and environmentally made, regarding media, and especially social media, not to forget the beliefs of the past feeding into the false narrative that disability is something to fear. This fear that society feels ultimately has a knock-on effect to people with disabilities, the isolation is a major contributor. If we carry on the way we are, this cycle of fear will be never-ending, and humanity will seize to develop on an intellectual standpoint. Humanity would be stagnant.

List of Hidden Disabilities

Here is a list of different hidden disabilities, disabilities that don't necessarily require a physical prop to confirm the fact. Admittedly, I'm a little apprehensive to list these different types of

Disability and Mental Health

disabilities, for the simple potential risk of having people who aren't disabled in any way, taking advantage on a very pressurised system as it is, therefore, potentially postponing much needed care to those who actually need it, ultimately jeopardising mental health further in the long run. Now who's being cynical right? I'm only being realistic, however. I'm listing these as a means to educate you. A means ultimately to decrease further judgement.

- ADHD

- Autism

- Asperger's Syndrome

- Personality disorders i.e. bipolar disorder, schizophrenia etc.

- Depression

- Anxiety

- OCD (obsessive compulsive disorder)

- Dementia

- Traumatic brain injuries

Disability and Mental Health

- Learning disabilities

- Diabetes

- Chronic pain or fatigue

- Respiratory conditions

- Incontinence

- Hearing loss

- Sensory and processing difficulties

- Multiple Sclerosis (MS)

- Myalgic Encephalomyelitis or chronic fatigue syndrome (ME/CFS)

- Visual impairment and limited vision

- Aphasia

- Asthma

- Renal failure,

- Sleep disorders

- Cancer

- Epilepsy

Disability and Mental Health

Really, any type of disability which inhibits daily life.

Listing every single hidden disability would be a book in itself. There are a whole host of different invisible/hidden disabilities to consider. All you have to do is research invisible/hidden disabilities on the Internet, and a whole list of these types of disabilities just waiting to be discovered.

For example, I'm adding in the link to the *Sunflower Scheme* page on their website which lists 900 hidden disabilities:

https://hdsunflower.com/uk/insights/category/invisible-disabilities

Inaccurate Symbol

My argument of the international symbol for disability, not being an accurate representation of all disabilities within Disabling Ableism is warranted here. A wheelchair isn't representative of all disabilities, it is really only representing a small number of disabilities. According to The *World Health Organization:*

"About 10% of the global population, i.e. about 650 million people, have disabilities (1). Studies indicate that, of these, some 10% require a wheelchair." – ['Fact Sheet on Wheelchairs', WHO (World Health Organization)]

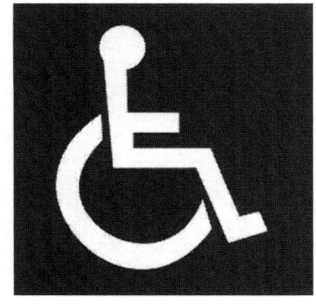

I'm covering old ground here I know, but having this symbol (left) as the accepted image for disability is outdated, and in many ways, offensive. With only 10% of the global population requiring a wheelchair, this is quite redundant to use this symbol as an identification of disability. As of Friday, 7th June 2024, according to the most recent United Nations figures, there are an estimated 8.1 billion people on the planet. This number is more than likely going to keep rising as the years go by, and yes, there will be a larger percentage of people who require a wheelchair if the population increases, this is inevitable, but the amount of people with disabilities that doesn't require a wheelchair will grow too. Equal

Disability and Mental Health

representation of these people needs to be improved and improved today. People can have numerous different types of disabilities that doesn't require a wheelchair. This image is only encouraging the wrong message, and misleading society to only think that a disability of any kind equals a wheelchair. I know that there are numerous other symbols for other disabilities (as shown right), but the above symbol is the main recognisable for disability somehow. The wheelchair symbol is internationally recognised, which is only perpetuating the wrong message that disability equals wheelchair. I believe that this is the reason why people in society have issues with different types of disabilities. It's been culturally ingrained and anything that goes against this learned narrative is alien.

On a side note, some accessible facilities now have a message to say that not all disabilities are visible (example left). I personally think this is a start, but so much more could be done to improve awareness of the fact. Just adding a small message to an accessible facility door, isn't really enough. Proper action needs to be undertaken. Again, it could come down to the simple thing of education.

Accessibility Symbol

A very good friend of mine, Jeff Dawson, (CEO of

1st Enable Ltd.) after reading my paragraph on this exact subject in Disabling Ableism, made me aware of a different image which is on most devices now, (right) which, in my own personal opinion,

really is a better representation of disability. It isn't referred to as 'disabled' either, but as 'accessibility'. This term at least to me, is much more encouraging and progressive. Since researching, I have been pleasantly surprised to see this accessibility symbol being implemented within a number of different websites, and devices.

As I've said before, the accepted image for disability is a person sitting in a wheelchair, but this image isn't representative of all disabilities. Not all disabilities are visible, not all disabilities require a

Disability and Mental Health

wheelchair. In short, this image isn't the best for the disability demographic.

Why Is This Identification Change Important and Relevant to the Progress of Mental Health Restoration?

Currently, a person with an invisible disability only has this one image to use, a person in a wheelchair. You hopefully can understand why my above comment is valid? The wheelchair image is an image that doesn't represent them at all. This instantly makes a person feel insignificant, unidentified and unsupported by society if you don't use a wheelchair, I don't need to have an invisible disability to understand this, this is obvious. Misidentification of one's own self could be put at risk. I know it's only an image to you, something that seems insignificant in the long run, in the grand scheme of things, but to a person who has a disability but isn't a wheelchair user, this misrepresentation can have detrimental effects. It's interesting what exactly can trigger a mental health issue, there are countless reasons. Being misrepresented in such an open way, is also a valid concern. You are ignored, judged, excluded. The audacity of this terrible mistreatment, so openly broadcast to society, and also subconsciously believing that this one image somehow is representative of a whole demographic. It so isn't. It's offensive if nothing else. That's the truth.

Other demographics are represented well today for the most part, admittedly you do still have comments (mostly through social media, because it's easier for these people, ('cowards' as I like to refer to them as, to hide behind a screen)). For the most part however, other demographics are being accepted and welcomed into society. It really is heart-breaking to me that disability doesn't get the same level of recognition, if at all.

In my personal opinion, the term 'accessibility' is far less daunting, and less label inducing than the terms 'disabled', or 'disability'. 'Accessibility' is welcoming, friendly, it's a better term all round. The 'accessibility' term helps to minimise ableism by subtly indicating where accessible facilities are, and also giving people dignity and respect. The word 'accessibility' doesn't necessarily shove the label in the public consciousness. The actual accessibility image doesn't scream 'disability' also. Of course, this can be considered both a good and a bad thing, but because the image isn't using a specific disability to identify disability as a whole, in my opinion, the good reasons outweigh the bad.

However, if there was an image change suddenly, would it be embraced as the wheelchair image has in public consciousness? Does the image have enough weight behind it to make a smooth transition? Is the image clear enough? Is it recognisable, or would the accessibility image ultimately be confusing? Would it be accepted? After all, the standard wheelchair image is the accepted disability image. Change can be difficult. Would people with disabilities feel more accepted or not? A lot of questions that can be overwhelming. The accessibility image itself doesn't necessarily give any disability identification after all. Some quick online participant research would be helpful here.

The 'Accessible' Afterthought

Everything seems to be a 'tick box' exercise with disability, there's no actual thought put into how to make things truly accessible. People think by just sticking a couple of grab rails on a wall, it's their job done. It's 'accessible'. It would be funny if it wasn't so sad. I feel that it's just done as an afterthought to please the powers that be. An 'accessible facility' isn't accessible just by putting a couple of grab rails in. There needs to be room for a wheelchair to manoeuvre, carers, a hoist, grab rails, things that make an accessible facility properly accessible. Having people with disabilities working alongside builders when building these accessible facilities would save a lot of time. I know of *Changing Places UK*, and the fantastic job they do, but for those public places without these facilities for one reason or another, I urge you to think on and act. You don't want to be seen as ignoring disability, do you?

Automatic doors are great, but they need to be built into every aspect of a building, I was at an event recently with my publisher Allan where they had automatic doors installed in one part, but none on the other. At another event, I was angry to learn

Disability and Mental Health

that the building used to have floor Braille for people with visual impairments to know where they're going, but during the revamp of the building, this Braille was removed to make the building more "aesthetically pleasing". The absolute definition of style over substance. Plus, the lift wasn't working I was told, because simply it "didn't affect the staff of the building, repairing said lift wasn't a priority"! It's disgusting.

This attitude only creates more turmoil, more angst for a person with a disability. Instances like this only proves the point that there is a problem. It can be mentally draining on an individual not being able to go about their daily lives just as everyone else, due to carelessness or prioritising style over substance. It can create a real mental health issue being denied access to life constantly. People may feel that they don't want to go out, in case they cannot access the place they want to go, so choose to stay in, creating more isolation and loneliness, and therefore, risk of further mental health decline. It's a slippery slope, but one that can be so easily avoided.

You may think I'm being dramatic, but it's true, and it should come from a place of wanting to make society more accessible, not just as a tick box exercise. Accessibility is a right, not a choice. By doing these things, it will create far less upheaval in the long run, and help those with disabilities feel welcomed into society, thus decreasing mental health deterioration.

Hidden Disabilities Sunflower (Scheme)

There is a dedicated scheme for hidden disabilities. It's the *Hidden Disabilities Sunflower*, also referred to as the *Sunflower Scheme*. Knowing that there is a scheme that represents the people in society with invisible (or hidden) disabilities, is fantastic, but is the scheme well-known to the general public? Does society know what the Hidden Disabilities Sunflower or Sunflower Scheme actually is?

"The Hidden Disabilities Sunflower is a simple tool for you to voluntarily share that you have a disability or condition that may not be immediately apparent – and that you may need a helping hand, understanding, or more time in

shops, at work, on transport, or in public spaces." – ['What is the Hidden Disabilities Sunflower?', hdsunflower.com]

You may have seen this lanyard (right) before? A green lanyard with a sunflower decoration. Did you actually know this lanyard is to identify those with hidden disabilities?

I conducted some quick social media research, asking this exact question, if people know what the lanyard means? I'm glad to say that everyone who answered, said yes, which is good to hear, but it does make me wonder why some signs on disabled facility doors have the 'not all disabilities are visible' sentence? Also, I do wonder if general society knows that proper understanding of hidden disabilities should be undertaken, rather than just taking it at face value, and whether this knowledge either helps or hinders a person's mental health who has a disability? I wonder if shops, work environments and transport are aware that the lanyard may mean that a person with a hidden disability may need a bit more time to execute a task, board or exit transport, and more time in shops, and in public areas? (Depending on the hidden disability of course). I may look into this at a later date, but it is definitely something to think about.

The lanyard really is a clear indication of hidden disabilities if research is anything to go by. Although, I completely understand that people with invisible/hidden disabilities may not want to wear the lanyard as it can be a blatant labelling mechanism.

This is the main issue I have with disability identification; you have to label yourself in order to say to the world that you may need assistance. Yes, it maybe voluntary, but if you don't wear a lanyard through choice if you have a hidden disability of some kind, then you can expect backlash. It must be easier to wear one in a way as a means to reduce potential backlash.

Really, all we are doing is just putting a sign on ourselves to say we're different. For me at least, labelling makes me feel instantly rejected as I'm seen as 'different'. Labelling for me gives society the false narrative that I 'don't understand'. That I'm 'vulnerable'. If those labels aren't there, this gives society permission almost to judge and manipulate, but in a different way. We need physical evidence to 'accept' a disability of any kind, and I say 'accept' in quotation marks, because it's clear that people don't really accept disabilities in the way we would like. People don't even tolerate disabilities in my view.

People just discriminate, but in a way where it isn't as obvious. The discrimination is constantly bubbling under the surface, and every now and again, the discrimination erupts like a volcano, but ends as quickly as it came, just enough to keep up with the pretence of an accepting world. On the other hand, however, I understand why people with hidden disabilities feel like they need a lanyard, it's to let people in general society know that they need help, and they require assistance, it's to stop any appalling and humiliating questions being asked.

"People living with disabilities that are not immediately apparent face distinct challenges

that significantly impact their experience of the world. Through greater recognition and accommodation of non-visible disabilities, we can foster a more inclusive and supportive society for all." – [Annette Cmela, Global Chief Brand Officer, Hidden Disabilities Sunflower]

It is funny to me how people with physical disabilities want to be treated as everyone else in society, when people with hidden disabilities, want to be seen has having a disability. Neither case is fault of the person who has a disability, fault, - in my own personal opinion, can be placed solely on how the world operates today. We have become so blindsided, so cynical, ready to call out things that go against our understanding. Yes, we have adapted our way of thinking to a degree in recent years, but this adaptation hasn't gone far enough in my opinion. Disability is still black and white. If you're disabled, you're a wheelchair user. That's the way of thinking. The reality is that a disability can be absolutely anything that limits a person's movements or ability to do things. This may sound counterintuitive to what I am trying to raise

Disability and Mental Health

awareness of, but in all honesty, a disability of any form can impact on a person's ability to do certain things in life, but this shouldn't be seen as a vulnerability, we shouldn't be treated any differently as a result. We are capable in most respects; it's about giving us the opportunities to discover those abilities for ourselves. Everyone is good at something. A person with a hidden disability has a whole other fight on their hands trying to be recognised for having a disability. This also can cause untold angst.

One person who answered my social media research on the Hidden Disabilities Sunflower lanyard was a social media participant who wants to be referred to as 'Diz', and who had a very interesting view about their lanyard.

"Yes, I am disabled, have used mine pre-COVID, when flying. So many non-disabled people started using them that I rarely use mine now." – ['Diz', social media participant]

It's interesting, yet sad that anyone would stop using their disability identification because it's ultimately being sabotaged by the general public. For me, I would completely understand if the reason was simply because of the labelling factor but reading that anyone would stop using the identification because others are taking advantage, is absolutely devastating. Nobody should ever feel apprehensive to use something designed for them. Society should never take advantage of people who have a disability of any kind and use these things for their own means. It's absolutely disgusting. It is also frustrating because people do think that disability is an 'easy option', but it isn't. Disability is a label, a minefield, filled with uncertainty, discrimination and prejudice, but society definitely does not see the negatives, even though it's usually society that instigates the negativity ironically. I can speak from personal experience that I feel disrespected when I see general society blatantly use things such as disabled facilities, myself.

For example, I was recently on holiday, and I needed to use a disabled facility, I had to wait for an adult with their child to use said facility. The adult didn't even know I was outside the door until they eventually opened it. The guilt on the adult's face was palpable when they saw me sitting outside waiting to use something designed for me. What kind of message does this send to the child? That it's okay to use a facility for quickness or if the female or male facilities are full? I 100% understand – 'Diz's' frustration, because it is really disheartening for people in the general public to constantly use something designed to make a person with a disability life easier.

Hidden disabilities arguably do have an unfavourable reputation. There's a collective misunderstanding and stigma towards hidden disabilities. Two examples of this misunderstanding that I can think of is how society reacts to disabled parking bays and public disabled facilities. There seems to always be a stigma, questions are always asked on a person's ability (or inability) when it comes to these two examples in particular. Unless you have a physical disability, you are unworthy of the label it seems, which is just depressing in all honesty.

"We often hear from people living with invisible disabilities how the lack of understanding from society is a barrier to access. When others make incorrect assumptions, it can create a sense of fear, upset, nervousness, irritation and frustration. These negative emotions can significantly impact their confidence to engage in everyday activities such as shopping, banking, travelling, and accessing pleasurable activities such as entertainment and holidays." – [Chantal Boyle, Communications Manager, Hidden Disabilities Sunflower]

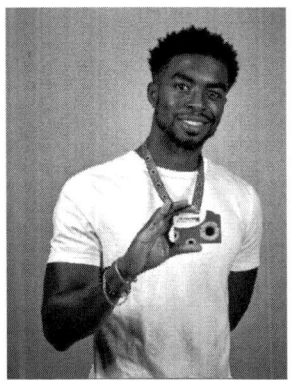

It's so sad that people with hidden disabilities often feel uncomfortable to live their lives, for fear of being judged for not conforming to disability standards.

Nobody should ever be made to feel terrible for their type of disability, as if they're an imposter. This

Disability and Mental Health

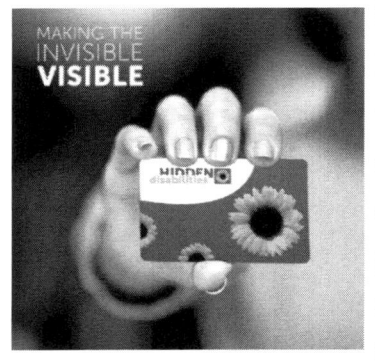

is just despicable. Nobody should ever be forced to explain their disability either, it's demeaning. After all, it's personal to the individual at the end of the day. Yes, there are those who play the system and lie in order to get the same 'benefits' as a person with a disability, both physically and fiscally. In a way, I can understand why society questions those who have either a hidden disability of some form and compares the person to what is understood to be disabled. It's to really protect those people with physical disabilities, as there are those in society who blatantly take advantage of disability. However, by questioning those people with hidden disabilities, this is blatant ableism and can create unnecessary stress and anxiety.

There is a *Hidden Disabilities Sunflower* lanyard available, (left), but I wasn't sure if society understood what the lanyard actually meant, so I conducted some quick social media research on the topic, and all of the participants knew what the lanyard meant. So, knowing this, a *Hidden Disabilities Sunflower* lanyard should be worn at all times in order to make it easier for society to identify. I do wonder however whether people with hidden disabilities do feel dehumanized by wearing the lanyard as it can be considered another label, another barrier in which will have to be fought against.

"...Hidden disabilities are often difficult due to society not seeing the disability, so making something visible does help. It's also not having to explain things." – [Rachel Williams, social media participant]

Rachel Williams, who uses one of these lanyards, said it best when she explained that having a *Hidden Disabilities Sunflower* lanyard makes it easier, as it makes a hidden disability more visible, so it is highly more likely that a disability won't be called into question. These lanyards are great for removing the need to ask personal questions. It's a quick identifier. It's a label yes, but to answer a

Disability and Mental Health

previous question, I can imagine wearing a lanyard is easier to live a relative 'normal life', without constant ableism. Society needs a physical prop in order to identify a disability. If this is what it takes, then so be it. I just wish that these props wouldn't overshadow the person, but unfortunately, they do. It's been culturally ingrained into society over the years that disability equals vulnerability. This is an outdated belief that should be erased to match with the modern world we claim to live in today. There needs to be more education on disability as a whole, but there also needs to be an emphasis on hidden disabilities in my own personal opinion. Hidden disabilities deserve to be recognised and respected. This respect argument needs to extend to disability in general also.

Mental Implications of Societal Advantage

You see some people in general society blatantly apply for disability benefits, as it's 'easier' than getting a job. Disability is treated as an alternative lifestyle. People only see what we have (which is very little by the way, opportunity wise) compared to the rest of the population, and often decide to try and 'become disabled' in order to get as much as possible. Nobody sees the other side of disability. The hardship.

There are invisible/hidden disabilities, granted, I'm totally aware of this, but everyone it seems do tend to jump on the bandwagon and try to take advantage of our disabilities by using and obtaining things which are specifically designed for us. It is evil, plain and simple. There's no other way to describe it in my own personal opinion. There's absolutely no excuse.

As part of the research, I asked Diz to explain their feelings when others in general society use the Hidden Disabilities Sunflower lanyard:

"A few years ago, there was an explosion of non-disabled people encouraging others to go pick up sunflower lanyards, and using them to get the accommodations we need, seeing them as perks. This made me furious, as those of us with invisible disabilities were often assumed to be cheats. I therefore stopped using my lanyard and other facilities, such as radar locked loos, for

years, apart from when I was flying. As this has calmed down, I use my lanyard more often, especially as I now don't go out in public without my walking stick or rollator, so I am more visibly disabled (eye roll). – [Diz, social media participant]

I actually went as far as to test how 'easy' it is to obtain a Hidden Disabilities Sunflower lanyard. All you basically have to do is fill out a form. There are no background checks or anything. I know that it may be done this way to prevent difficulty for the person actually needing the lanyard to order one, but in reality, this also means that anyone can cheat the system and lie in order to obtain one for themselves. This isn't me just speculating either, there's actual evidence of this happening from 'Diz's' comment.

You also see it with Radar Keys now. I've covered this in Disabling Ableism, but a Radar Key is essentially a key for people with disabilities to use a disabled facility. These keys are only meant to be used by a person who has a disability. Nobody else in society should be able to possess one. Before, to obtain a Radar Key, a person with a disability would have to apply for one from their local council and there were checks put in place to make sure that you met the criteria of disability. Today, anyone can get a Radar Key on the Internet. Bypassing checks. You have the capability to just order a Radar Key from a shopping website or even on the high street. Why the method of getting a Radar Key was made easier, I don't know. Maybe it's the same possible reason as obtaining a Hidden Disabilities Sunflower lanyard? Which is good in theory, but as already established, making things easier for one, will also make things easier for others. Government needs to remember this before any decision and action is undertaken, which will affect those in society with a disability. This in my own personal opinion only adds to the misrepresentation of disability. We are seen to have an 'easy life', with all of our benefits, our perks, in reality however, this couldn't be further from the truth, and definitely needs to be recognised and rectified.

I for one, feel angry when I see others in society clearly cheating the system. It makes me, and I'm sure others, feel disheartened and angry. It shouldn't be possible to get anything without proper checks. I feel misunderstood and depressed in a way to think that general society blatantly disrespects disability. I for one, cannot fathom why anyone would want to claim to be disabled when they aren't. Disability isn't a lifestyle choice, it's a part of life. You don't have respect, independence, equality, nothing like this, it is an uphill battle just to be recognised for who you are as a person, and equally hard to be recognised as being disabled if you have a hidden disability. No matter how you look at it, disability isn't an easier alternative at all.

Label Focused

Disability is just an invitation for ignorance. Society cannot see past the label. Society is just focused on the label, that they forget the most important thing, the person.

With this obsession, people with disabilities can become indifferent to themselves and start to hate themselves because of their disability. This is what eventually happened to me. My mild Cerebral Palsy became the be all and end all to those in society, that it started to affect my self-esteem to the point where I hated what I saw in the mirror. The beginnings of this self-hatred started in secondary school. I thought when I started, it was because I wasn't 'fashionable enough', so I tried to alter my appearance to try and 'improve' my overall look, but the bullying I experienced was solely down to my physical disability. I realise this now in hindsight.

I guess pupils didn't want to be seen with me as this would ruin their own social life, their reputation, but there's absolutely no doubt in my mind that the mistreatment I experienced in secondary school, shaped me as a person through the rest of my teenage years, going into adulthood and the majority of my 20's.

This mistreatment wasn't an isolated case unfortunately. It became apparent that my disability was going to hinder my chances of finding employment. After graduating, I had extremely bad and degrading experiences in employment which ultimately contributed towards my own mental health deterioration. Being fired from jobs, not

Disability and Mental Health

being given any work, being manipulated and lied to alongside many other unfathomable experiences, hit me hard. I became a shadow of my former self. All of this negativity which I personally experienced was due to my mild Cerebral Palsy. This was the main reason why I had so many negative experiences.

I craved attention, and so, I became a people pleaser, trying in vain to get noticed and wanted by a certain employer, but they saw this need in me to be wanted, exploited it and took advantage, which only meant I fell further into this need to be accepted. It was a never-ending cycle that just plagued me mentally and emotionally for years.

Nobody understands that a person with a disability can develop mental health issues in response to the mistreatment that comes with disability it seems. I can't help but wonder whether if society took the time to understand the connection between disability and mental health, whether the discrimination and ableism would stop for good?

Although, sadly, something tells me that the mistreatment wouldn't stop. We will just have to put up with it until the end of existence and be okay about it.

Chapter 4
The Attraction to Stay Silent with a Disability

People with disabilities aren't heard, that's the long and short of it. Opening up about your mental health if you're struggling, letting yourself become the possible target for further backlash, ignorance and ridicule, on top of the ableism we almost always face, isn't really an attractive prospect. Staying silent if you're struggling with a mental health issue of some form, alongside having a disability, you may think will stop you from becoming an outcast of bigger proportions, but ultimately, that struggle will materialise in some way, whether you choose to try and hide those dark feelings away. Believe me, I know all too well.

This was my logic when I was personally struggling mentally. I didn't want that for myself. I didn't want to be known as a "disabled person with mental health issues", already being known as a "disabled person", or an "object" was bad enough, without

The Attraction to Stay Silent with a Disability

adding my personal struggles into that mix. I was fighting to be recognised as a person first as it was, not just as a disability, but I was also fighting a personal mental battle. My mental health issues mainly stemmed from the discrimination that I faced, so I didn't want society to find a reason to discriminate me further, if that makes sense. So, I chose sadly to stay silent, thinking that I could manage the struggle alone. I became that 'actress', performing just to get through the day, letting the 'true me' at the time manifest at night, when nobody was around to see.

However, this fight of trying to manage my mental health issues, whilst also 'acting' ultimately contributed to my mental health deterioration ironically. In the end, staying silent is what became my downfall.

A mind can only take so much.

Every single negative experience related to my disability I faced, only added to that pressure cooker. I thought that I could handle it on my own, and I believed that I was good at pretending. What

The Attraction to Stay Silent with a Disability

I hid in the day, I 'dealt' with late at night, often by eating a load of sweet things, and crying into a pillow, muffling the sound in case I woke everyone up. I thought that I had everyone fooled. They all knew. My main family really. I was only fooling myself. At some point it was obvious that it was going to come to a head. I understand that now. I kept a lid on my struggles for so long, years in fact, that the pressure cooker just exploded one day. My head couldn't take the burden of carrying the heaviness I placed upon it anymore. I thought that I could keep a handle on it, that eating a mountain of chocolate throughout the day and night, crying into a pillow, was going to solve my issues. It may sound strange and implausible to you reading this now, but at the time, my mind was just so far gone from where it once was, rationality wasn't top of the agenda. 'Coping' was.

I say 'coping' and 'dealt' with quotations, because obviously the way I chose to 'cope' and 'deal' with my personal struggles, my inner turmoil, wasn't 'coping' or 'dealing' with the situation at all. If anything, my methods were only putting a sticking plaster over a bigger issue.

Deliberately Stopping Questions

"Other kinds of silence might be empowering. Some with mental illness are defiantly silent because the people around them ask unwelcome questions or give them unhelpful input. They might wisely choose to save difficult conversations for their therapist. Such a choice isn't necessarily rooted in stigma." – ['Mental health: It's not always good to talk', Dan Degerman, University of Bristol]

Describing the act of choosing to stay silent as 'empowering' is quite interesting, yet alarming to me at the same time. Yes, opening up can be overwhelming and frightening, there's no denying this. The way Dan Degerman puts this down to society, almost blaming society, can have a potential danger of blocking people from seeking proper support. There's a danger of mass scepticism, alongside a potential social divide, which of course, isn't great for maintaining equality.

The Attraction to Stay Silent with a Disability

I get Dan's point however, but this point can be mistaken as to believing people are just unhelpful. This may create more mental health deterioration in the long run, as those with a mental health issue may purposely hide their feelings away more, thus creating a bigger issue with mental health decline. A catch 22 situation.

I absolutely understand the logic behind the statement, but we need to start being more optimistic with important topics that can have a detrimental effect on a person's life. Please don't take that optimism term out of context though. Being too optimistic isn't healthy. We sometimes need pessimism to balance things out. What I mean when I say about being optimistic with important topics is really, not to shy away from them, but embrace them. Society needs to start being more open and willing to learn about ALL important topics, including mental health and disability, we can't just pick and choose what topics we embrace. To be fully inclusive and equality driven, all important subjects that have an impact on society needs to have the same level of attention. Only

The Attraction to Stay Silent with a Disability

then, can we truly be a modern world, and just not claim to be.

For this scenario to have any weight behind it however, mental health needs to be at the forefront of the minds of the population. This is the job of Government to make sure that important topics are highlighted properly.

You have campaigns now such as *ITV's 'Britain Get Talking'*, which is a step in the right direction, but there obviously needs to be more of this type of awareness if Dan Degerman's statement is anything to go by, there's still an issue with people potentially not opening up about their mental health issues, for fear of simply not being understood.

There is also the fact of pride. Someone who is struggling may feel a sense of humiliation if they let people know that they are struggling. It's the curse of pride. There are so many areas and reasons as to why a person who has mental health issues opt to stay silent, paint on a smile and try to carry on that false 'happy' life. The life we want, and more often

The Attraction to Stay Silent with a Disability

than not, deserve, but a life that is so far removed from our reality. This knowledge can severely damage our mental health further, depending on the level of our mental anguish. It's a catch 22. You're damned if you speak up and damned if you don't.

Given that the above quote from Mind is from 2015, thankfully, media, (at least), have got this memo on the importance of maintaining our mental health. I will cover this in plenty more detail in a later chapter.

How have we got to this point where ignoring our mental health issues are better than confront ng them? It's just unreal how we think avoiding is better than facing up to the issues. It speaks for how society deals with their issues in 2024 as of writing this, it may have changed by the time this book is eventually published, but – (and I hate to be pessimistic with this, unfortunately, however, I fear that I'm only being realistic) – I really do¬'t think anything will have changed for the better, given the quote from *Mind* in 2015, nine years ago, again, as of writing this. Needless to say, this is a real problem.

Silenced

So, why have I named this book *Silenced*? The reason is actually very simple. Mental health issues can be a struggle for many, regardless of cause. People generally find staying quiet whilst going through difficult times the easiest option, but alternatively, people with a disability may feel they are forced to stay silent and tow the line to what the label is understood to be.

There's also a sneaky second reason for the title, I deliberately haven't mentioned the word disability, or any word related to it, to make it more appealing to society. Am I deceiving you? Only you can make that conclusion. It's up to you, you can stop reading here and continue to live in a world of social deception, or you can continue and learn how to make the world more equality driven. Yes, I know my books are heavy, but how disability is mistreated is equally as heavy, if not heavier. As people with disabilities, we live in a world where

The Attraction to Stay Silent with a Disability

deception rules. Pretending we are equality driven on the surface, whereas in reality, it's anything but. In a sense, I'm giving you a taste of that deception in the hopes of changing it for good.

There is more awareness of mental health today and keeping a check on us and others around us generally, thanks to campaigns etc., but it still can be difficult to open up to people if you're struggling, as you may not know how or where to start the conversation.

Similarly, there could be a temptation to stay silent for fear of being bombarded with unwanted and unhelpful questions. You may not want to be associated with mental health issues for the feelings of shame or being looked at or treated differently. Sympathy often comes with the territory of having mental health issues, you may not want to become that vulnerable person, especially if you are seen as a strong, fun-loving individual. You may not want to tarnish that image of yourself forever.

Also, depending on your situation, hiding your mental health decline, you may believe, is essential to help you progress. Stress can bring on mental health issues. Higher education can be stressful and challenging as you constantly chase deadlines and may have revision etc. The pressures higher education can create are intense. Education in general as a whole can be a stressful time anyway. Body image, popularity, bullying, revision, exams, and exam results can also cause stress and mental health deterioration. Then there's the everyday stresses of work, unemployment, money worries, bills, etc., that can plague an individual.

PTSD

Of course, mental health issues can also develop as a result of a traumatic event, and so PTSD (Post Traumatic Stress Disorder) may develop as a result.

"Post-Traumatic Stress Disorder (PTSD) is a condition that some people develop after experiencing or witnessing a traumatic life-threatening event or serious injury... Anyone exposed to trauma can develop Post Traumatic Stress Disorder -...PTSD sufferers can have many 'triggers' – sounds, smells, tastes, things you see,

and the emotions you feel can all bring back the trauma, presented as real life – a flashback." – ['What is Post Traumatic Stress Disorder?', PTSD.uk]

As a direct result, people who suffer from PTSD may avoid speaking about their trauma as an attempt not to be reminded of it.

"This usually means avoiding certain people or places that remind you of the trauma or avoiding talking to anyone about your experience." – [Symptoms – post-traumatic stress disorder, NHS.uk]

There are many potential reasons, and therefore, a silence may begin, as a failed attempt of 'copirg'. Again, I say 'coping' in quotation marks because people who stay silent whilst struggling with a mental health issue of some kind doesn't 'cope', they just act. Act without getting any recognition or payment. This is the hardest job of all.

Keeping Up with The Pretence

The Attraction to Stay Silent with a Disability

Pretending to be happy when you are not can be difficult for anyone to master. You have to summon up the energy and the courage to be able to do exactly that, and finding the motivation to do so is harder when you have a mental health issue, especially a mental health issue which is caused by society, but you do it.

You simply don't want to be asked intrusive questions that can ultimately label you further. You need help, but terrified of being judged further. It's bad enough that your disability automatically labels you. You don't want to give society an excuse to discredit you more. So, you push those feelings of self-loathing down deep inside, you plaster on a smile and adopt a happy demeanour just to avoid further barriers. Yes, mental health is getting the recognition it deserves, but disability doesn't, marrying the two topics doesn't seem to register in the minds of society. There's this disassociation between the two somehow? Maybe out of fear? Maybe out of ignorance? To be honest, either or indeed, both reasons could potentially be the case, I just don't know. What I do know is that this

The Attraction to Stay Silent with a Disability

misunderstanding leads to further mental anguish. It also goes against what is believed that a person with a disability should be happy, and grateful all of the time. There is a resilience to stay silent with struggles anyway, especially with the male population. It is that fear of being stigmatised for the rest of your life still, even though mental health awareness is commonplace today. There's still that reluctance to speak out. What chance does disability have with this mentality?

It's ironic to me that people in the general public fear being stigmatised and labelled if they take the brave step to speak out, yet, this is what a person with a disability faces every single day, with or without a mental health issue. It's usually the mistreatment of disability in general society that cause mental health issues, by in large.

Of course, there can be other significant factors that can contribute to mental health decline, if you have a disability, and you may feel ashamed to admit it, such as the self-loathing, especially but not limited to developing a disability later in life. Pride is often a factor in this case. You may not want to

The Attraction to Stay Silent with a Disability

tarnish your image further by admitting a mental health issue has developed alongside your new way of life. I can imagine that it can be a harder thing to adjust to anyway, you don't want to appear weak on top of everything else. Developing a disability later in life, I cannot begin to imagine the turmoil this can present.

Then there can be people who have a hatred of themselves because they have had a disability all their lives. Seeing other non-disabled people doing things when you can't, can be frustrating and devastating. You want to be like them, but you can't. You're stuck in a broken body that cannot work the same way. People see you and make assumptions of you off the bat without asking. So, you can retreat into yourself, becoming depressed. It can be harder to make friends because of the silence, which makes you even more depressed and hate yourself even more. It's a never-ending cycle.

Although not the exact same reason as above, I became self-loathing and silent in secondary school. Yes, preschool was a factor to my trauma, (the beginning of it if I'm honest), but secondary

The Attraction to Stay Silent with a Disability

school was a whole new kettle of fish that I had to endure. I talk about this more in the next chapter.

Silence can be a choice, or it can be a response, but ultimately, staying silent when you have a mental health issue of some kind regardless of who you are isn't healthy, nor does it help you or others around you. I learned that the hard way. It's tough I know, I've been there, I know what it's like. You know you need help, but you want to be left alone at the same time. It's horrible, but unless we take that first step then we will just continue on the path of self-destruction. I know it's a cliché, but unless we help ourselves, nobody can help us. Talk to someone, a close family member or a friend. It doesn't even have to be someone you know. There are helplines out there such as The Samaritans and Mind that can really help, even charity's which specialises in disability can help such as, Scope, Sense, and Mencap. If talking isn't your thing, then writing can be an option. I personally have found writing a safe have. Before writing, I couldn't see a way out. There wasn't a light at the end of the tunnel. I was just constantly existing, not living.

The Attraction to Stay Silent with a Disability

Everything I tried to do for myself came crashing down around me. The moment I started writing, everything fell away. I was no longer burdened by my past. I took back control. It was cathartic just writing everything down letting people know what I went through without actually having to verbalise it. A real weight was lifted.

If you have a disability or not, the importance to speak out is crucial to social understanding. I do wish there was more information about disability and mental health out there, but not written in a patronising or stigmatising way. Mental health on its own is becoming a part of social consciousness now, but disability is still on the backburner, and knowledge of disability related to mental health? This is virtually non-existent.

I urge Government to look at this as a serious matter that urgently needs to be addressed. Although I'm not expecting this plea to be recognised sadly, as I'm only one voice trying to raise awareness of disability equality and mental health, but it would be fantastic if there was any action as a direct result of my writing. The recent

The Attraction to Stay Silent with a Disability

bill is hopeful, but I hope it's just the beginning. I hope that other areas will be looked at and reformed, such as making disability education essential in all areas of education and the workplace. I've been lucky enough to deliver talks alongside my publisher Allan on disability education in colleges and universities, and the response has been phenomenal. It just goes to prove that disability education is welcomed, it just needs to be implemented properly.

I'll be honest, it's wonderful to work with Lesley Griffiths, MS for Wrexham on a couple of projects recently to enhance disability inclusion, alongside speaking with the Mayor of Wrexham 2024-2025, Counsellor Beryl Blackmore about disability awareness. My hope is that they read this book and decide to help me raise awareness further with the impact of mental health in relation to disability.

Then, and only then, can we start to see real change, which could help end the silence forever.

Chapter 5
Mentality vs Conformity

Ultimately, it should never have to be this way. Nobody should ever have to conform to social ideals. Everyone is individual after all. Nobody is made the same way. This lifestyle often plays into potentially devastating effects on one's mental health.

Everyone has different strengths and weaknesses. This is obvious written down on paper, right? It makes sense. You know you. You know what you can do, and indeed, what you can't. Disability or otherwise, you just know your limitations, and nobody wants to be told their limitations in whatever capacity. That's just ignorant and rude. Choosing what **you** want in life without anyone else deciding for you, should **always** be enough to live a relatively independent lifestyle. It should be paramount. Again, the bill is testament to this. You should be genuinely encouraged – (not encouraged out of sympathy or empathy). You

Mentality vs Conformity

should have people who genuinely want you in their lives, either in a social or a professional capacity, and do everything that they can to make this a reality. Discouraging isolation and promoting inclusion. This is what should be happening. The world isn't like this, however.

Why? We live in a world of conformity.

"...the process whereby people change their beliefs, attitudes, actions, or perceptions to more closely match those held by groups to which they belong, or want to belong, or by groups whose approval they desire..." – ['Conformity', Britannica.com]

We, (as a society) are forced to conform. It really doesn't matter if deep down we don't agree with certain things, we almost have to adapt our way of thinking to match others in society. Our thoughts aren't our own. We crave approval from others every single day. It's addictive, like a drug. It is the way of the world nowadays. If you don't look or act a certain way, you are instantly the outcast, because it has been trained within us, that everything that goes against the 'norm' is alien to us. We have this uniformed way of thinking. You do see individuality starting to peek through, albeit with the help of *Pride* as just one example, helping to build better relationships in society, but you still do get the odd look, the odd comment from certain people in society who are just set in their ways, and only see a blinkered viewpoint of life. It is mostly a generational thing admittedly. People in the past were brought up to believe certain things, and this way of thinking has carried through to today's way of thinking. Moreover, with media and especially social media creating tension and hatred constantly, these certain people do in a way, get their views validated.

With a certain type of generation, it's not enough just to say something isn't PC (politically correct) anymore, there just seems to be a passive attitude when this term is mentioned. Often laughed and brushed off. This though is exactly why a conversation with subsequent action needs to happen. This conformity stems from a combination of the past, and indeed the present with

Mentality vs Conformity

technology picking up the attitude of the past but accelerating it.

Race, gender, and homophobia are the biggest issues that poison technology, our online world, but one issue that seems to go under the radar for some reason is ableism. I think it's because ableism isn't directly interlinked with society. Society can choose to ignore disability as it doesn't really affect other people. It only effects the person with the disability, so it doesn't matter if we ignore those people who have disabilities, as ultimately there will be little to no backlash. With other subjects like race, sexual orientation, and gender, to take three examples off the top of my head, these are more integrated into society, so more noticeable. Rightly, there's a chance of getting called out for online hatred and abuse of race, homophobia and gender, admittedly, not all of the time, but there's a chance. There doesn't seem to be an issue with ableism, because it isn't in your face 24/7 like the other subjects, all of the other subjects do tend to get more media coverage today, but disability does seem to be on the backburner. I feel this is why disability does seem to get the brunt of the abuse and/or ignorance, because it isn't as widely known as it should be. There are virtually no news coverage on disability, and for what there is, it's either bad or positive, but not positive in a good way, patronisingly positive, like it's amazing someone can do something as mundane as I don't know, getting fantastic exam results, but because of the disability, that disability tends to outshine the actual achievement with the focus being more about the person's condition, the disability becomes part of the news story and takes over, for example:

"Sam achieved 6 A stars, despite her disability."

Then the piece may go on to say more about the person's disability rather than what they've done to achieve such grades.

I hopefully don't need to tell you how awful that is? This is what I mean when I say that people do seem to be obsessed with disabilities. Imagine being judged, labelled, patronised, every single day of your life. Always being told *"No, you can't"*

Mentality vs Conformity

because of a disability which is insignificant compared to the actual person. Frances Ryan shared something very telling recently from *X* formally *Twitter* about the *2024 Paralympics*. A non-disabled commentator said:

"You stop seeing the wheelchair pretty quickly when you watch this sport."

To the untrained eye, this may seem like a good thing, but personally, as with the person who posted this and with Frances Ryan, I take issue. A wheelchair isn't a part of the person, a wheelchair is a **mobility aid**. Something to get you from A to B. You wouldn't say this to a driver of a car, but because it's out of the 'norm', it's fascinating? Why? There's absolutely no rhyme or reason to say things like this, if you do, you're only adding more fuel to the fire, maintaining the stereotype.

Societal Conformity

People in general society may be tempted to conform to social ideals by joining in with unfounded beliefs just to 'fit in'. People may not believe or even understand what they are conforming to, it may just be a tactic to become a part of society rather than feeling like an outcast. In a way, it's a form of peer pressure. The ironic thing is, this pressure to socially conform to stop you from feeling like an outcast, ultimately may make others with disabilities for example, feel like the outcast. This can also make a person with a disability want to conform, believing if they go along with the narrative of how disability is perceived, then maybe they'll be better treated? I really don't know the logic here for why a person with a disability may want to conform to the 'idea' of disability. Maybe because they are sick and tired of trying to alter perceptions, that they just surrender to it, as it may be easier to do so in the long run? It seems that if you aren't willing to conform to social ideals, you are instantly ignored, you're unworthy of being seen as more, and when I say more, what I mean is you are unworthy of being seen as yourself. If you have a disability of some form, you are only recognised by your disability, the biggest hidden barrier that a person with a disability faces every single day.

Mentality vs Conformity

There is only so much a person can take. You do get to a point where you actually think "what is the actual point?" Nothing is working to end the stigma. You may as well just surrender to it, because this is what society thinks of you anyway. The incapable, vulnerable person. The label. It is extremely depressing to come to this conclusion if you have worked hard to have the same opportunities as everyone else in society. You just lose yourself to the idea of disability in the end.

This is known as conformity bias.

Conformity Bias

Again, with how reliant the world is on technology (which will be covered in more detail later), there is a real issue with conformity bias in society. This conformity bias can be linked to ableism, as currently, disability is generally seen as a negative, especially on the Internet, so in order to try and improve public image, there may be a pressure on a person with a disability to conform to the idea of disability conformity as it were, as an attempt to fit in. Personally, I'm guilty of this myself in secondary school, doing everything I could to fit in, but it was useless as my wheelchair was always there, reminding people that I was 'different'.

Conformity bias is dangerous and detrimental to the whole population, as it lends itself to obsessive tendencies. General society may adopt conformity bias as a means of trying to fit into the crowd too. It doesn't mean to say these people actually believe in what they are doing, they may just be doing it to be part of general society.

Conformity bias doesn't just affect a certain number of people, conformity bias affects the whole world.

Chapter 6
The Statistics

Statistics arguably aren't respectful, especially if those statistics give information about sensitive and important topics like mental health, as it only groups people together, removing humanity. However, statistics can be useful for projects such as this. However, even though these are statistics, please remember that each statistic is a person first and foremost, a living, breathing person. Statistics only add to the invisibility and detachment we automatically have when statistics are involved.

General Society

The statistics on general society's mental health deterioration is as follows:

- **Mixed anxiety and depression: 8 in 100 people**

- **Generalised anxiety disorder (GAD): 6 in 100 people**

The Statistics

- *Post-traumatic stress disorder (PTSD): 4 in 100 people*

- *Depression: 3 in 100 people*

- *Phobias: 2 in 100 people*

- *Obsessive-compulsive disorder (OCD): 1 in 100 people*

- *Panic disorder: fewer than 1 in 100 people.*

[Information from Mind.org.uk]

These statistics are worrying, yet unsurprising, given how the pressures of life are more magnified today. Life today is extremely pressurised. Life today is extremely fast paced. To accompany this extremely busy lifestyle, everyone and everything are put under a metaphorical microscope. People with disabilities generally have this level of mental anguish heightened, because of that disability factor. Everyone is judged, and as a result, judgemental of themselves almost every single day. We have to fit in a box, conforming to social ideals.

We cannot be individual. We have lost this ability as time has gone on.

A person with a disability has everything decided for them, because it's believed, (wrongly by the way) that if you have a disability of some form, you're unintelligent, and so cannot have independent thought. It's telling that if you have a disability, your independence is taken away from you so much in an instant, that our right for independent thought is also affected negatively. It happens, because of course it does. Yes, this unfortunately has happened to me in the past, and sadly, it wasn't an isolated incident. It **never** is when disability of any kind is involved. It's the 21st century after all. Our attitudes should have improved towards different areas of life, but it needs so much more improvement. Yes, it's improved over the years, but it's obvious, (to me at least) that more could be done to improve disability awareness and inclusion.

It's frustrating and anger inducing. We are silenced, hence it being a struggle for many who live with a

The Statistics

disability of some kind. We are just **expected** to shut up and put up.

For many, relying on others can be extremely demeaning, dehumanising, depressing and hurtful, but because of the disability factor, these feelings annoyingly get ignored. When you've been independent all your life, it can be a real shock and defeating to accept. This can be for a whole host of different reasons and feelings.

- Undignified
- Dependency
- Pride
- Surrendering
- Vulnerability
- Labelling
- Weakness
- Fear
- Guilt
- Self-hatred

176

- Disrespect

Media has taken hold of us, and we are destined to conform to what is 'acceptable' by media standards.

The reality is extremely different because of conformity. We are continually forced to conform to social ideals and understandings of disability. If you have a disability **of any form**, usually, once either of those terms are mentioned (disability or disabled), that's just the end of the road. Those negative perceptions of you start to develop, regardless of who you are as a person. People have preconceived ideas of disability, so you can have the mentality to succeed, the determination, but as soon as either term is mentioned, nobody wants to know anymore. A disability trumps a strong mentality, qualifications etc., every single time. We cannot challenge, or educate, we just have to sit on the side-lines and watch whilst others in society take your success, and it's all because of some insignificant thing that has absolutely no bearing on the **person**.

The Statistics

Admittedly, there are those who don't realise that they are being patronising when they are in the presence of a person with a disability, but in my own personal opinion, this complete lack of knowledge is actually worse than knowing. If you are unknowingly being ableist, then it just goes to prove that sadly society is being brainwashed into thinking that disability is equal to vulnerability, that it's something negative, and the narrative that this belief is okay, which of course it isn't on any level.

This belief partly comes from how disability was mistreated in the past, coupled with the 21st century, with all of its technology, social aspects, and information (often misinformation in this regard). We are happily sleepwalking into this conformity and ever growing ableist culture. Isn't it time to change negative perceptions into something positive that would ultimately benefit both the people with disabilities and non-disabled in the long run.

Now, I do know the potential reason for resistance here. By rule, society often learns about the subject of disability, (especially today) harshly, society has been taught and ingrained into culture. The overall consensus is we are incapable pure and simple. It's almost as if this is just the accepted image and description of disability. To being taught this, you are only setting up to fail. To have this one, blanket description your whole life, suddenly change, then of course it would have somewhat of an effect on you. After all, your belief system has been externally altered.

The option to stay silent after such rejection and conform to the idea of disability can be seen as the easiest path to take in the long run. The idea of just existing is better than being scrutinised in many ways. It's not worth the hassle. We aren't respected for who we are, we are just seen as this label and should just go along with the narrative.

I know this, and please bear in mind, that I'm just going by my experiences at this point, as this has happened to me in the past, especially whilst job hunting after graduating from university. The negative impact that rejection had on my mental health at the time, was a lot to deal with. I grew insecure with myself. My confidence plummeted so

The Statistics

much. It got to a stage where I didn't see the point in trying anymore. I gave up on everything, myself, my family, potential employment, just absolutely everything. I basically just decided to give up. Nobody respected me or my achievements, so why should I have any shred of self-respect?

Nobody actually realises the potential negative impact their actions can cause a person. Society thinks that words are enough, but unless those words are then backed up by genuine action, then it's not modernisation, it's patronisation, ableism and deception. I did self-harm for a while. Yes, this sounds cliché, but I guess I just wanted to feel something, instead of always constantly feeling numb. I'm not ashamed to say it now, that was a dark period in my life that did take its toll. The rejection and ableism I suffered from society encouraged my thought process at the time. I started to believe that I was useless, incompetent and vulnerable. Even though I just graduated from university at the time, whilst dealing with personal trauma of my late nan, Mary and my lovely little dog, Bubbles both passing away during my time at university, which didn't matter one little bit. My wheelchair trumped everything, my qualifications and myself. There's only so many times a person, regardless of who you are, can get back up after being constantly knocked down. The fight in you slowly vanishes, and you get to a point where you just give up, and let the negativity flow, you can't do anything to change people's minds, so what is the point? If you carry on trying to fight for what you want, your self-esteem is going to get significantly worse because nobody is listening to you. You are just trying to shout over a soundproof cement wall as it were. It's useless.

Not A Modern World

We aren't a modern world, we cannot be, if things such as what I personally went through still happen.

Needless to say, this is the main issue I have when people claim we live in a modern world, because it's clear we don't. A modern world, (especially in employment) is accepting and willing to give people opportunities if they are qualified and want to work, regardless of who we actually are.

The Statistics

Employers desperately need to reverse their beliefs, because their beliefs, - I can guarantee you – are formed either entirely, or in part from other influences. Our thoughts aren't our own. We rely on others to tell us what we should believe in – I digress here, I will come back to this later, but this unhealthy mind set, (because it is unhealthy by today's 'modern standards') encourages our mentality to decline, both as in potential mental health issues arising. A strong mentality should never be dampened or belittled. It should be celebrated and encouraged. Our disabilities shouldn't be celebrated or encouraged when that celebration and encouragement is only due to sympathy or empathy.

A modern world wouldn't use conformity. A modern world wouldn't use patronisation as a conversation tactic when talking to someone with a disability. A modern world wouldn't have groups specifically designed to belittle and humiliate those who have a disability. None of these examples would happen, but unfortunately, they do, and one place conformity happens are in disability groups.

The Problem with Disability Groups

I know this as I've seen it happening, and actually have unfortunately experienced this situation many times. I had to take part in these types of groups, where proper communication is at an all-time low. I actually was recently invited to one of these groups (as of writing this), - a long story as to why I attended. Let's just say for now that the people caught me under false pretences. Again, I was promised something that wasn't real. It makes me wonder why people who organise these groups think it's a good thing. These groups only enhance the stereotypes and ableism, as we are categorised as one demographic. A group for disabled people? It's just conformity at its best. Our mentality often doesn't match our physical appearance.

Again, not to discriminate against those with invisible/hidden disabilities, but in this type of scenario, a physically disabled person often finds it harder to disassociate themselves with their disability as the physical 'prop' is there to remind society of that disability.

The Statistics

Disability groups from my personal experiences only cater for a specific type of disability, and so, the activities are often degrading and demeaning. Staff in these groups patronise and belittle those who join. The issue is, because the staff who run these types of groups have a certain type of disability in mind, they just cater to that one type of disability, without realising that not all disabilities are the same. Do people realise how their actions affect others in general? It really does annoy me because this wouldn't happen in general society, but because disability is seen as the weaker demographic, thanks to media, we somehow just have to 'deal' with it because we look a little different? How is this fair?

Personally, I have absolutely no issue with a disability group which is specifically aimed at young children with a disability, having activities that usually are for preschool age children, as this would be a specific type of demographic. When you reach the ages of 10 to adulthood, this is when a disability group should think of those attending, and in my opinion, cater the activities to those people. A 'one size fits all' approach doesn't work. It's demeaning, degrading and just abhorrent to see these disability groups not moving on and realising that other people who are arguably more capable than others deserve to be treated as an equal. It's the blatant disrespect that I take issue with. A disability group can be a fantastic thing, but frustratingly, they aren't thought through properly. Assumptions are made, but these assumptions only make those on the receiving end feel labelled, judged, feeble, branded, insignificant, ignored and discriminated against. Those with high mental capacity feel misrepresented and so this misrepresentation can have detrimental effects. You get to a point where you feel like what's the point of trying to be seen as more, as obviously, it isn't working if disability groups are even labelling me? You do get angry. You think to yourself that you've worked hard, and you are only disabled physically, this shouldn't have any bearing on you as a person. Disability for many wrongly also means you are unintelligent. How? A physical disability doesn't always mean that. I mean yes of course there are

The Statistics

those who have both a physical disability and a learning disability, **BUT NOT ALL**.

We need to get out of this mind-set of ignorance. We need to start seeing people for who they actually are, people. We should accommodate to people's abilities, not assume. By assuming, you are taking away our control, our freedom of choice. Forcing people without learning disabilities to play pass the parcel, paint by numbers, see child friendly films in the cinema etc., is just wrong, plain and simple. It just plays into the false narrative. There should be age-appropriate activities for those people who don't have learning disabilities but attend these groups. Staff who run these groups should look at their members and realise what would be beneficial activity wise. Again, I completely understand that there are those whose mental capacity is low, and would benefit from activities that are deemed easier, but for others there should be a choice, and an actual choice, not saying that an activity is being organised and just giving you the choice of what you want for lunch. No. Full control is needed.

These groups are a label all on their own, but they don't need to be.

Chapter 7
My Own Struggle

Admittedly, I wrote in depth about my own personal experiences and struggles before, especially in *CP Isn't Me*, so if you wish to read a bit more of my time in secondary school and the world of work, you can in *CP Isn't Me*. However, for the purposes of this book, I intend to give an overview of the experiences, with an in-depth focus on how those experiences made me feel at the time, and how those experiences make me feel today with hindsight.

I've concluded that when you're at your lowest ebb, downtrodden or just appear vulnerable by appearance alone, this is when people like to take advantage of you or your situation, gaslight you, or deny you, just to see you drop further into turmoil and despair. We live in a society where nobody cares about anyone but themselves, (main character syndrome), people take advantage of others and situations for personal gain. This is how society has

My Own Struggle

been brainwashed. This behaviour is toxic to mental health. In a way, for humanity's sake, this is where the pandemic was crucial to reverse this selfishness, everyone said we needed to get back to how we were pre-pandemic, which was true virus wise, but I argue that we need to return to how we were behaviour wise during the pandemic. Egos were demolished, everyone was on equal footing and kinder during this time. That's what we need to get back to, kindness and understanding to lessen mental health issues for **absolutely everyone in society**.

With every negative experience, every denial, every ignorant comment, every patronised word, just every time I was subjected to emotional and mental abuse solely based on my disability, another little bit of me died. I felt like I didn't belong anywhere, that everyone I met and interacted with hated me for what I was. People refused to see me, just me, without the wheelchair. The wheelchair was, and often is the biggest antagonist for me, I mean, not as much today since becoming an author, but there are still instances of ableism in my life. It's crazy to me that in order to have any type of respect, I've had to address my past so publicly. It has served me well, I'm not denying this, but it seems that a person with a disability of any kind, always has to prove their worth in some way to have any type of chance. If you have a disability of any kind, proving yourself is difficult. It's like a cement wall and you're trying to tear it down with a teaspoon. You're not worthy of opportunities, your path is chosen before you can decide, nobody will listen or help, you're just stuck in a situation that you can't escape from. It's horrible. Often, in most cases, you just feel ike what's the point of living anymore? It's blunt anc to the point, but it's true. You get to a point where you don't have any fight left. That's what it felt like for me at least.

Preschool

This is a time in life where you should be taught, feel safe, and encouraged. A young mind is still learning about the world around them. Children are trusting. Adults have a responsibility to ensure that young children are getting the information needed to learn about life. This though as established in *CP*

My Own Struggle

Isn't Me wasn't the case sadly. My experience in preschool was anything but pleasant. In a word it was traumatising, and I am **not** describing the experience as this in order to gain attention or for you to feel sorry for me, I hate being patronised, sympathised and even empathised, despise it actually. I'm just telling my truth of how I felt back then. It must have affected me badly because I can still remember every single horrible detail of the situation which, I believe, gave me trust issues for life.

Power should never go to someone's head, especially if you are working with young children, but this is exactly what the person did daily. A standard preschool day lasts for a couple of hours, but when you are forced to sit in a wooden chair, facing a wall with a window, taunting you with the sunny outside world every day, when you're sat in a dark, depressing building, crying for your mum to come back and save you, is obviously going to be traumatic for anyone, let alone a young child with a mild form of Cerebral Palsy, like me, is somehow worse as it's blatant ableism. The person in charge was really a tyrant in watching me suffer. I believe they actually enjoyed seeing the turmoil. I know that the person didn't like me, but I didn't like them either due to their mistreatment.

This was the first time I was exposed to the real world. The mask slipped drastically. It wouldn't surprise me if I developed my trust issues then. After this experience, that darkness followed me. It also makes me wonder if what I was feeling was a form of PTSD? It was diabolical for me, and remember, a couple of hours feels like a lifetime as a child, especially if you are being discriminated against. You have no concept of time as a child. An adult should never bully any child. The person hated me because I was nervous and scared of my own shadow. I refused to participate in activities because basically I was terrified. In hindsight, I'm not sure why I was like this, there was no reason feel that way, I had a fantastic home life, with a loving and supportive family, I guess I was just scared of certain things.

If you work with children, as previously mentioned, you should be understanding and encouraging, you

My Own Struggle

should never segregate a child, but this is exactly what happened to me on a daily basis. I used to scream not to go because I knew what was waiting for me. I remember the gut-wrenching feeling. I remember feeling sick to my stomach, shaking with fear, pleading not to be taken there. At that age, I thought I was being punished and I didn't know why. I felt that I was going to be abandoned there. I thought my family didn't want me anymore. As soon as I saw that building, my heart rate accelerated, I started to hyperventilate, I couldn't breathe. Just writing this down now, I can still feel the panic set in, even though I'm in my early thirties now, so, you can imagine how the preschool mistreatment negatively impacted me in later life?

The person in question did absolutely nothing to help me, if anything, they only added to my distress. They lied to my family, just saying that it was separation anxiety so my family believed this, why would they question it? Separation anxiety is a genuine thing, but being so young, I couldn't articulate what was happening, all I could say was I didn't want to go. My family only had this and this certain person's theory, and they put 2 and 2 together. I was a nervous wreck by the time my parents decided to take me out of preschool, I felt so alone, I physically and mentally felt drained when it stopped. I remember that. I was glad to leave, to get away from that monster, but the whole experience left me feeling down and scared of starting a new school later in life in case I was mistreated again.

All I'm going to say is my family finally found out what happened whilst I attended that preschool, and they couldn't be sorrier. It wasn't their fault though. They thought it was just separation anxiety, and they trusted the person in charge. I definitely don't blame them at all. If you want to read more on this, more information is in *CP Isn't Me*.

In today's world, I really don't think that this experience would be allowed to happen. Today, there are many checks and safety procedures put in place to help prevent things like this happening to others, which obviously, is extremely important.

My Own Struggle

Secondary School

This can be a difficult time for anyone. Navigating through this environment full of judgement and scrutiny can have detrimental affects on mental health. You almost have to be equipped to deal with potential issues that can come with secondary school both in an educational and social capacity.

If you have a disability of any kind, well, unfortunately you are already identified and treated differently. You are the 'disabled kid'. This is you for the rest of the school time. This is your label. You don't matter to anyone. You are automatically judged. If a non-disabled pupil is bullied because of their appearance, then you have a choice and chance to change your appearance, of course, nobody should have to change their appearance in order to try and improve their social status, (I can imagine that this would be flagged up today, considering how awareness of identity is at the forefront of society nowadays – this is ironic to me, how is it that we can accept and support identification, but disability is still controversial?) Why is disability still mistreated by society today, given how other subjects are arguably treated more humanely? How is this fair?

As I've mentioned before, as a child, my own disability wasn't an issue for me really, or anyone else for that matter. I think because as a child, you aren't as effective or active in everyday society. You exist yes, but you aren't actively going to find work etc. Hence, you don't actively participate in everyday society in the way in which you would do as an adult. I virtually had no real issues that affected me as a child, other than my time in preschool.

As soon as I hit the age of secondary school however, people's perceptions of me significantly changed for the worse. From then on, I was on a downward spiral. It was as if I was enemy no. 1. My confidence deteriorated, that's the long and short of it.

I was bullied in secondary school, and yes bullying is a part of school life, but disability does add an extra obstacle between pupils in a secondary school environment, this is because the stakes are

My Own Struggle

higher in secondary school. Image and popularity are everything. There's a hierarchy (which admittedly is silent), but the judgement is there. My secondary school did run on segregation, making it harder to mix. There was a constant feeling of isolation and loneliness. Every single day I was made to feel inadequate to the other pupils in the school. The pupils with disabilities were compared with the mainstream school. I wasn't any different from anyone else, but it was the wheelchair, the physical prop that blocked me from being seen as anything other than my disability. When I was in secondary school, we weren't allowed to go out on the yard with the other pupils at break times or lunch times, we were forced to sit in a room altogether with a support worker. We weren't even allowed to participate in sports days. We had to sit and watch other pupils participating in sports days. Compare this with my experience in primary school where I was allowed to go out on the yard with my friends at break times and lunch times, and we were allowed to participate in sports days.

My Own Struggle

In secondary school, we were treated exactly the same, as just one package. It didn't matter our intellectual abilities; our physicality came first and foremost. Our disabilities were our identification, we weren't. Do you know how belittling that is? How anxiety inducing? Personally I was a shadow of my former self, crying every single night for what would've probably happened the next day. I was a nervous wreck. It doesn't sound like much, but believe me, unless you actually lived the experience, it won't sound like much. Being told that nobody loves you, wants you, that you're a burden, alongside more hateful things related to suicide, having doors slammed in your face, eating lunch alone, having support workers 'find friends' for you, being whispered about, pointed and laughed at, being segregated, having support workers themselves gossip about you to other staff in the school, wouldn't you cry every single night?

We were treated as insignificant. So, we were compared with others, knowing that we couldn't do anything to match the expectations, and so, we were ignored, tossed aside, made to feel inadequate. This attitude was very visible to me, but I couldn't do anything about it, because nobody would listen to me. My opinions and feelings didn't matter. Image mattered, and not only to the pupils, but the staff too. It was extremely annoying. It made me angry. I mentioned previously that the staff would give us all a warning beforehand, rules to abide by in order to get a good report when inspections were due. We were forced to mask the school, give it a sickly-sweet image. Almost being the advertisement for the school. This ironically was the only time where disability equality became a part of the school. We were trolleyed out, put on display. For a week, we were treated humanely, being allowed to go out on the yard with the other pupils in the school, and being tolerated by those other pupils, just to appear more inclusive to the outside world. You could argue that this was a great week, but I, like others, knew the truth, and besides, a week would soon end. As soon as that Monday after inspection week rolled around, you can guarantee that those changes would automatically be reversed. The mask slipping to reveal the true nature and beliefs that the school held. I felt physically sick every single day.

During this time, I withdrew within myself. I became quieter, timid, crying every single school night for what lay ahead the next day. It wasn't a school, it was a prison, the disabled pupils were the prisoners, and the non-disabled pupils and staff were the prison wardens.

The only relief, the only respite I had was on a Friday at 4pm, when I got home for the weekend, and lasted until Sunday evening at 10pm, when that exponential dread of the next day would immediately set in as soon as I went to bed. To reiterate, I did have insomnia during this time, I never slept a wink. Needless to say, I had several panic attacks. I was struggling.

It was a silence.

I was silenced by the school, struggling to cope every single day I attended. How can this be allowed?

My Own Struggle

To give a bit more context on the seriousness of the situation, some support workers took great pleasure in belittling me by discussing my private life outside of the disabled toilet door of all places! How ridiculous is that!? It was also extremely unprofessional. It was unpleasant, and it affected me quite badly. The trust was gone. To be fair, I had very little trust in that school for anyone to begin with, but any shred of trust I did have was quickly removed once that horrendous time period began. I wasn't respected by pupils or staff (mainly support workers – 2, possibly 3 that I can think of, made my secondary school experience worse, simply by acting like the pupils, and spreading gossip.) I was angry, but also hurt when it happened, I was at a complete loss. I wasn't myself anymore, that happy-go-lucky kid with loads of friends, with no trust issues, disappeared. All of that was gone. I was gone. In that once happy person's place was a cynical, depressed, highly emotional human being who was constantly lonely. I tell you, if it wasn't for my brother Ian, taking me on numerous different outings after school during this period of time, I just know that I wouldn't have managed. I arguably wasn't coping well anyway during the day, but I regret to imagine what I would have been like if I didn't have Ian, especially during this dark time. Ian reminded me for one night every 2 weeks, who I once was. I had a glimpse of my old happy life; it felt fabulous for a few hours. I could forget the issues school provided for a few hours, and replace it with fun, joy, and laughter. I wished those nights would last forever. I needed to escape my reality. Ian did this for me. Thank you once again Ian, I'll never forget what you did for me. You saved me. I love you.

Looking back now at my time in secondary school, I actually feel bad for the non-disabled pupils in a way, not completely however, because even though staff in the school during this time could've set an example, children at this age should be more aware and equipped to handle different situations independently, but again, I feel because of the social media presence having a hold on society today, sadly, we have lost the fundamental principles that makes a just society, and by extension, **every staff member should have** (especially in a school environment), leaders. Leading by example, showing respect and therefore, gaining respect. This unfortunately didn't exist when I attended at least. Staff members (and especially the pupils) made that school in particular, a living Hell, to put it mildly. I was defeated, we all were defeated. We were targeted, the joke. There wasn't a way out, as time went on, the mistreatment got worse, being verbally abused, and sometimes physically abused. It is well documented by now that I personally had doors slammed in my face, which was awful for me. To go from being popular in primary school with many friends, to then exchange this for abuse and loneliness, was a jarring experience which I wasn't prepared for at all.

Work

Today, I'm extremely happy and content with my working life, honestly and truly, (and when I say work, I still mean volunteering), but the difference is, I know for a fact that both my new bosses in my Tenancy Support and Social Media Developer role, alongside my job as a graphic designer for a local acting company, actually genuinely appreciates and cares, they aren't just saying it to sound good, as they've said as much. I have regular check-ups, meetings, given a lot of trust of which I truly appreciate. Given how I was mistreated in the past during my working life, it really is a refreshing change, and I couldn't be more thankful. I see now how you **should** be treated, compared to how I was mistreated and controlled in the past. I was coercive controlled in one job I had, I see it now. The rose-tinted glasses have finally been surgically removed, alongside the weight in my mind. These certain employers never really cared, they just saw an opportunity and ran with it. Promising me the Earth, but not delivering, gas-lighting me into thinking that it was all in my head as to why there was radio silence from them. These certain employers would praise me when I went to work, couldn't do enough for me in fact, but as soon as I finished for the day, that was it, no contact. It was if I didn't exist. They loved the power they had over me. Like as if they were dangling a carrot in front of a hungry donkey, but instead of letting the donkey

My Own Struggle

have the carrot, they would take it away, making the donkey crave the carrot more to the point where it would do absolutely anything to have it. Yes, I'm aware I'm the donkey in this scenario, but it's true. Everything they did was only go have a sense of power over me.

These new voluntary job roles tie in extremely well with the subject matter with my books which is wonderful.

I go around houses the charity organisation purchases, then adapts in order to make the accommodation more accessible to people who benefit from the service. I go into these accommodations to see if they are truly accessible or indeed not. This is progressive, because this is what I truly believe, and probably said before, that publicly accessible facilities should always be designed and built by involving people with disabilities, asking their opinions and suggestions on how to make the facilities **truly** accessible. The public should ask the disability demographic in question, then I can guarantee you that there wouldn't be as many issues. This is what should be happening across the world.

This new job is perfect, given what I write about. Not to mention my volunteering as a graphic designer for the acting company. I'm finally holding the cards, and I absolutely love it!

It's safe to say that I haven't had the best experience of work up until this point in all honesty. The negativity revolved around my Cerebral Palsy in one way or another, such as literally being fired, being manipulated, getting ignored. All of these experiences obviously had a negative impact on my mental health. I lost who I once was, and the experience of working was the straw that broke the camel's back. I know that I said I was happy with a particular job, and I was, but I also think that happiness was surface level in many ways. It picked me up. It gave me purpose. It gave me an opportunity when nobody else would. Something of which I will always be grateful for. With my role as a Tenancy Support Officer and Social Media Developer however, I feel that I'm truly making use of all my talents.

My Own Struggle

I used to feel useless, empty, unappreciated, insecure, untalented, depressed, anxious and needy. If you are mistreated, fired, unsupported, oppressed, exploited, and disrespected throughout your working life over the years with your different jobs, if they have helped in your mental health deterioration, then of course you're expected to feel insignificant.

I've been in situations before where I've literally had to beg for work, or other employees of a company have had to give me work to do, as a certain employer in particular was 'uncomfortable with my disability', and so couldn't bring themselves to speak to me like a human being. I felt like a monster. You shouldn't have to beg for work or have other employees of your company give you work to do. The working world shouldn't work like this. It's unethical and discriminatory. It's absolutely a degrading situation to be in, needless to say humiliating. You feel insecure and isolated. Why should this be allowed? If a non-disabled person experienced this level of disrespect and discrimination, then I can guarantee you that the world would definitely know about it, because it's in the mainstream. It's public interest. News and media in general would chomp at the bit to cover the story, for ratings if nothing else.

I know it's not exactly the same, but as an example of a news story that would gain interest is the recent closure of *TATA Steelworks* in Port Talbot, Wales, which has been covered extensively since the announcement of closure back on 18th January 2024, jeopardising 3,000 jobs in the process. It's devastating obviously for the former workers of *TATA Steelworks* with regards to loss in income and supporting the families of the former workers. This has made national news, and don't get me wrong, it is extremely important, and of course the mental health of those former employees, must be rock bottom at the moment, but I really can't help but think if a story revolved around ableism, would get the same level, (if at all) of attention? It's wrong yes, but it's also reality unfortunately. Disability isn't as impactful as general society's issues. It's not as newsworthy. It's not relatable, and this is the issue.

My Own Struggle

Work and disability never seem to register. It doesn't go together. We are weak, how are we able to maintain a job? It's an oxymoron, but is it? This belief is solely based on hearsay, what is written down, what's in the public domain, but it's not reality. Capability is based on the individual.

A Ticking Time Bomb

This has been said before during this book in particular, but when you are constantly exposed to this mistreatment day in – day out, then it's so obvious that a mental health issue may materialise in some way. Depending upon how you are 'dealing' with everything, it maybe difficult to see your mental health deterioration. It could be subtle to you, whereas it could be obvious that there's a change in your personality to others, such as family and friends for example. It's easier looking at it from the outside. When you are a part of it, you can be oblivious to the fact. The mind is extremely complex that if you are in a continuous negative environment, it can numb you to the point of ignorance. It's that ignorance that actually gets you in the end. Believe me, I've been there, done that, got the t-shirt for definite.

During the ignorance phase of a mental health issue, I can describe it as a ticking time bomb, as you aren't addressing the problem, you are just ignoring it in the hopes of eliminating it, but by ignoring it, you're ultimately making it worse, This is ironic I know, but unless you've been in this situation you really have no idea.

For me, really, (as previously mentioned during my time as an author), it was a combination of close family members passing away, including my nan, Mary, my granddad, Irving and my 2 aunties, Christine and Julie, all passing away in quick succession from one another which added to the deterioration of my mental health, (and that isn't even including the passing of my dog, Bubbles and even Michael Jackson), which in context, sounds ridiculous, but unless you're me, you really have no idea how those two experiences impacted me mentally for years. Until my family members died, I didn't realise myself how much the loss of Bubbles

My Own Struggle

and Michael Jackson actually negatively affected me until years after.

Add ableism to this heartbreak, starting in secondary school all the way up to your late 20s, then you get a new type of psychosis. It's ironic to me that I experienced an everyday occurrence like death, as stupid as it sounds, but also having ableism thrown in there for good measure. It's doesn't make sense how I had to 'deal' with grief, but also 'deal' with ableism. I experienced both worlds and at one stage, at the exact same time. It's so sad. It was so detached from my feelings, yet I was in tune with my emotions, it was a strange period of time for me. I was living 2 lives, a non-disabled person's life, 'dealing' with grief, and a life of a person with a disability 'dealing' with ableism. For many people in society, the everyday stresses of life cannot impact on disability. I'm living proof that this belief isn't true. The pressure I felt, especially in my head was immense. It was a ticking time bomb and every negative situation I experienced, was just another thing to chip away at my sanity, until I eventually had that mental breakdown.

The Label – Others

I can tell you that others who I've spoken to or interviewed for my books have disclosed to me that they hate the words 'disabled' and 'disability', as like me, choose not to use the label to identify themselves, and honestly, why would you? Think about something about yourself that you aren't keen on, now imagine being identified as this one thing every single day of your life. It isn't that great is it? Welcome to our world.

Chapter 8
The 'D' Word

As established already, disability is a label all on its own that we have to unfortunately deal with daily.

In *Disabling Ableism* I spoke about Apartheid, and how really, Apartheid hasn't been eradicated, we have just swapped one demographic out for another. We have just replaced race for disability. Apartheid was about segregation. Segregating people based on the colour of their skin, which today, seems abhorrent. We wouldn't dream of doing anything like this, except we do, we segregate people with disabilities. We dehumanise people with disabilities, disabilities are mistreated just as race was mistreated back in the day. We treat disability differently to general society. There's segregation as already mentioned, but there's also many other things, hidden barriers if you will, which can seriously negatively affect mental health.

I'm going to ask you directly now, as a non-disabled reader. This is a genuine question. How would you

The 'D' Word

like to be mistreated every single day of your life? Being segregated, patronised, judged, labelled, manipulated for no reason whatsoever. Decisions are made for you. You aren't independent. You're unintelligent. You cannot do anything. You're said "no" a lot. It's really frustrating because these things shouldn't happen. We should be able to participate in society if we're willing and able. A disability should never stop a person from success. Ambition exists with every living person on the planet. That 'D' word, however, makes life harder, not for the actual disability, but the perception of disability. We are automatically put into a box, wrapped in metaphorical cotton wool. We don't live, we just exist to play the part, the idea of disability. The term poses negative perceptions on the public. It's a negative term, but sadly, it's not even your fault, you have been taught by outside influences over the years to believe that with a disability, a person is incapable to do anything. Disabilities are helpless. I think this stereotype comes from how people with disabilities were mistreated in the past.

"...Taken in total, throughout the ages, people with disabilities have been subjected to infanticide, starved, burned, shunned and isolated, strangled, submerged in hot water, beaten, chained and caged, tortured, gassed, shot, sterilized, warehoused and sedated, hanged, and used as amusement." – ['Psychosocial Aspects of Disability, 2nd Edition', Springer Publishing Connect]

Obviously, the mistreatment isn't as bad as it once was, as indicated above, but reading this myself whilst I was researching, it just made me feel sick to my stomach to learn how disability was actually mistreated in the past. I knew about the circus acts with 'The Greatest Showman' – (and I use this description extremely loosely by the way), PT Barnum, who categorically mistreated people with disabilities in order to gain a profit, (more about PT Barnum is written in *Disabling Ableism*), and of course, being placed into institutions if you were disabled, but I really didn't know how the mistreatment was inflicted until now. Disability or otherwise, how can one human being, treat another human being with such torture? People with disabilities were seen as less than human, this is why. We were inferior compared to the next non-disabled person. Bottom of the food chain, lowest of the low.

You may think at least this physical treatment has been abolished, and even though it's a small improvement, this belief still happens to this day. Nobody cares about the mental implications of disability mistreatment as it's hidden. There are no physical scars, but physical scars, even though abhorrent, heal. It's much harder to heal mental scars.

Disability isn't well represented, especially online. People generally make assumptions about others who have a disability of some form. I asked people to explain their own experiences of living with a disability and some of the negatives they have faced from people in society.

Rebekah Sims, has Ankylosing Spondylitis:

"Ankylosing spondylitis (AS) is a long-term condition in which the spine and other areas of

the body become inflamed." – ['Overview -Ankylosing spondylitis', NHS.uk]

Alongside Rheumatoid Arthritis:

"Rheumatoid arthritis is a long-term condition that causes pain, swelling and stiffness in the joints. The condition usually affects the hands, feet and wrists." – ['Overview Rheumatoid Arthritis', NHS.uk]

Rebekah also uses a wheelchair. It's important to note before you read her experience, that her conditions do not necessarily mean incompetence. Of course, this goes for all disabilities. This is her experience:

"It is more so the perception of others. For example, I was returning an item at the store. Instead of being asked if I have the receipt on my phone I was asked "do you know how to take a picture with your phone". It went from assuming I knew what it was doing to assuming I knew nothing at all. If I wasn't in the chair, she wouldn't have said this." – [Rebekah Sims, social media participant]

The 'D' Word

I cover this frequently in my books, but assuming that you cannot do things just because you may have a disability is again, ableist. I think people believe they are showing concern and care, but what you're actually doing is just adding to the negative perceptions, the stigmatisation. Why wouldn't we know how to use our phone? Just because we have a physical prop to indicate a disability. The discrimination that happens here is so comically blatant. It's just absolutely ridiculous. This behaviour by the public only encourages the notion of disability equals stupidity.

Rebekah's experience isn't an isolated case unfortunately. I've experienced the same assumptions. I asked Rebekah to explain her feelings after her encounter:

"It made me feel dehumanized. Like how could I not know how to download a receipt? And why did she assume I didn't know how to do that? In that moment I wasn't the badass woman with a master's degree who could do anything.... And I'm so confident too that's the hilarious thing.

But it took me down a few pegs for sure." –
[Rebekah Sims, social media participant]

I can unfortunately relate to Rebekah here. The lack of confidence. The dehumanisation. The loss of identity. Personally, it makes me quite angry that society can only connect disability with incompetence.

Another participant, Ian Jarvis shared his experience with living as a C6 paraplegic, and the challenges he has faced from people in society, alongside the subsequent effects on his mental health:

"What I discovered was that if I'm with someone and we go anywhere most people talk over my head to the person I'm with rather than me. It's often, though not always as if being in a chair gives the impression that my mental acuity must be diminished. Very often if I'm at an event and considering a purchase I'll roll away because I've asked a question, and the stall holder will answer whoever is with me rather than myself. However, if I'm on my own I suddenly seem interesting as

though it's a surprise that I function very well on a mental level. For me this was really hard to come to terms with because I've always been independent so to suddenly be treated as less than a full person really knocked my confidence."
– [Ian Jarvis, social media participant]

This is exactly what I mean when I say that disability has this negative attitude. It seems that you are either seen as 'vulnerable' or 'amazing' that you can understand the world. There's no in-between.

Assumptions are automatically made before you interact with a person who has a disability of some form. Why we are stigmatised is anyone's guess? Society is so obsessed with the narrative of the 'dis', that they completely ignore the 'ability'. We are seen as incoherent. People in society have done the exact same thing to me, talking to another person I'm with rather than me. It's frustrating to say the least. For a person who has become physically disabled during their lifetime, it must be crushing. To go from a confident person to constantly being belittled at every turn, must be a shock to the system. It's difficult enough if your disability has been with you since birth. Going from a person that society respected, to being patronised and stigmatised? I cannot begin to imagine the psychological pressures that this may cause.

If you are subjected to this constantly, it will eventually eat away at you until you become the exact thing that people 'think' you are. You become that vulnerable person, who is open to ridicule, scrutiny and sympathy. The label is one you cannot fully escape, no matter how much you try. It is your responsibility to ensure that you are different from others it seems. It's your responsibility to ensure that you conform to what it means to have a disability by social standards. Disability is seen as a negative, and anything to challenge this perception maybe met with confusion or even backlash.

A person with a disability is supposed to be 'vulnerable'. We aren't meant to be successful or be coherent. This goes against what society has learnt. Society cannot believe or fathom if a person with a disability of some form achieves something. There's usually a big fanfare that accompanies the achievement. I will speak more on this soon.

Chapter 9
Factors

If you have a disability of some form, there's a high chance of mental health deterioration due to public reactions and other factors. I'm going to list these factors within this chapter and explain why these factors can contribute to developing potential mental health issues.

Environmental

Environmental challenges consist really of inaccessibility. This is the main environmental challenge which can cause barriers between disability and general society. Buildings with no access, technology which is inaccessible or not adaptive etc., are just some examples of environmental challenges.

"Being wheelchair bound is filled with challenges. While we are thankful for the accommodations available, there are so many supposedly accessible accommodations that are

anything but accessible. Restrooms, small tight corners, hotel beds in accessible rooms being so high that a person cannot transfer from a wheelchair. I feel that all approval processes for accessible provisions need to be actually planned and approved by a truly disabled person." – [John Pam Lloreda, social media participant]

Disability presents its own set of challenges, John, has kindly given some environmental ones, which are frustrating because these are challenges that shouldn't be a thing in the 21st century. Accessibility for all should be commonplace. It's a basic human right. It's not a privilege, it should be standard. It's not a difficult request. More often than not, we seem to be denied life.

"...issues, including accessibility, can sometimes make someone with physical health issues more vulnerable to additional stressors or barriers. For example, problems with access to transportation could increase social isolation or keep someone from accessing services or employment, and this could further aggravate mental health problems." – [Richard Luke,

Specialist Information Officer and Cerebral Palsy Programme Lead, Scope]

Inaccessibility ultimately gives the illusion that a person with a disability is unable, but I argue that if society isn't accessible, well, of course we aren't going to be able to gain access, not because we are vulnerable, but because society isn't aware enough to make the world fully accessible.

It's like a non-disabled person not being able to access a locked room, because simply, the key to the locked door is lost. How frustrated would you be if accessibility (which should be commonplace), isn't actually there? Now, imagine that frustration dialled up to a million, and you still wouldn't be close.

The problem is, non-disabled people are hired to design and create 'accessible' facilities as John Pam Lloreda alluded to in their comment.

Things can be so much simpler if full accessibility was a reality in all areas of life. I've been in buildings with no lift, only steps to enter and exit a building. Yes, a manual wheelchair seems the best

Factors

solution to the untrained eye, but if the person with a disability cannot self-propel as I can't, this can cause lack of independence as you may need someone with you just to make sure that you can gain access and leave a building accordingly. This shouldn't be accepted though; a manual wheelchair cannot be an acceptable option. It's a lazy 'solution' more than anything. You wouldn't ask a person to walk a great distance if there's a road closure, no, there's usually a solution, a diversion, in order to prevent difficulty to get somewhere. Life doesn't stop for the general public, there's always some kind of solution ready to be put in place if there's a threat of disruption for society. For a person with a disability however, this isn't the case. Inaccessibility gets overlooked quite a bit when it comes to disability. Lack of independence anyone? Ableism anyone? The mental health implications this rejection can create is unnecessary and cruel. Inaccessibility can also come in the form of social discrimination, which will be covered in the next section.

Usually, having others with you if you have a disability of some form gives society permission the option to assume that you are vulnerable and as a direct result, may patronise you.

It is better than it was, but as John said, there are still issues in terms of accessible facilities, and even the height of beds in hotels in accessible rooms, if you don't use a hoist when getting into bed, trying to manoeuvre yourself safely is virtually impossible. It's actually dangerous. I wholeheartedly agree with John, there should be opportunities for those with disabilities to design and assess accessible facilities, rooms etc. These things are supposed to make our lives easier by creating more independence, but most things truly aren't fully accessible. How does it make sense for non-disabled people being allowed to design something that they really don't understand? This can have a detrimental effect on a person with a disability. All of these environmental challenges make us feel ignored and isolated, (speaking from personal experience), as if we are bottom of the social hierarchy. As if we don't matter. We are not accommodated to the extent

Factors

we should be. This is one of the barriers that ultimately block us from fully participating in society. This is when feelings of isolation, loneliness and abandonment can occur. Inaccessibility is ableism. In my own personal opinion, inaccessibility should be reviewed by Government, and not by assessing public areas themselves, but by asking those in the know, people who live with inaccessibility every single day, their views and suggestions on how to make society more accessible, and therefore, inclusive. We need action to be taken.

The reputation of disability is effectively tarnished within the public eye. Asking intrusive questions won't do any more damage surely? I can well imagine that this is the justification for using ableist language.

Social/Societal

Then, there's the social and societal issue, where assumptions fly all over the place when a disability is acknowledged, (or not as the case maybe). I'll discuss this further in the next chapter, but this again is unwarranted societal behaviour.

"...I have had strangers say things to my girlfriend, things like why you don't push him, had people ask her if she is my career and literally talk like I wasn't there, which as previously stated, just exasperate my issues of self-image. I would find after days out that I would have 2 to 3 days of depression, as being out in public would really make me feel bad about myself and feel like I'm not good enough for my partner, or that she could do better." – [Ben Ashby, social media participant]

This is what the general public doesn't realise I feel, the mental anguish their actions and words can have. It's devastating to me that people make others question their own worth, and in some cases, their life. This makes me angry that society can have the power to make a person feel insignificant enough to develop mental health issues, and the ridiculous thing is, society often is so ignorant to their own ableism, that they may not realise their behaviour is creating such angst.

Factors

Developing a mental health issue on top of all this blatant ableism is a very tiring prospect to contend with in itself. After all, you are battling so much that is concerning something that should never be a concern in the 1st place. Introducing mental health issues alongside the battle really isn't the best approach for so many. We are considered vulnerable as it is, knowledge of a mental health issue will only ultimately add to the vulnerability. People with disabilities are treated as second class citizens compared to the rest of society. You may not want to hear or accept this as fact, but unfortunately it is a reality. True equality wouldn't have environmental, social and societal challenges. True equality would **never** have a person question themselves. True equality is acceptance, no matter who you are.

I discussed in chapter 3 about the connection between disability and mental health with the quote from *Sense*. Mistreatment of disability is obviously going to take its toll if exposed to it constantly. Disability mistreatment is a daily battle, so of course those with a disability are likely to develop mental health deterioration. Sadly, it's inevitable. I have first-hand experience of constant mistreatment due to my disability, patronisation, manipulation, judgement, and just overall discrimination I unfortunately faced on a daily basis from the age of 11, right up until I was around 28 from numerous different sources. That's a long time that the mistreatment lasted for me. I'm lucky, I don't really get mistreated now, due to the fact that I'm now an author. People seem to respect me more and treat me as a human, and not just as a statistic. This shouldn't have to be the case. Nobody's worth should have to be proven. Everyone in the entire universe is good at something, but not everyone in the entire universe is good at everything. This is what society needs to understand and accept. Being identified solely as a disability and not as a person is crushing. It's soul destroying.

We are always perceived as unintelligent, as if we don't understand everything going on around us. Often, we are spoken about, not spoken to. If we have a non-disabled person with us, others in

Factors

society tend to ask them about us, not ask us about us. We are the best person to ask about ourselves. We know who we are inside out. If you want to know anything, just ask us directly. I think people tend to ignore us as they think they may offend us if they ask us questions. Questions are great! They break down those barriers. Not asking us questions about our disability directly is offensive.

As Richard Luke hinted at in his comment in the environmental section, inaccessibility can also come in the form of unemployment. I covered a bit about this in *Disabling Ableism*, but employers do tend to perpetuate the stigmatisation of disability. There's an unfounded assumption that hiring a person with a disability can cause so many other knock-on issues. It's in *Disabling Ableism*, so I know this as fact, but employers tend not to hire a person with a disability because they may the ridiculous assumption that the employee with a disability may have more time off, compared to other non-disabled employees, due to illness or appointments. The truth is, hiring a person with a disability can make the business. A person with a disability is dedicated, they work harder to prove their worth. Now, hiring a person with a disability and realising this fact, can be looked upon as exploitation. There's a fine line that needs to be realised. There are those who exploit others who are considered 'weaker' by social standards. I know, as I've been subjected to this myself, but for the most part, employers tend to steer clear of potential employees with a disability in favour of a potential non-disabled employee. It doesn't matter your qualifications or experience, more often than not, employers opt for the 'lesser of two evils', the potential non-disabled employee.

There's a lot of 'red tape' with a potential employee who has a disability. Hiring a person with a disability can potentially mean making the work environment more accessible, which in turn means spending money. It can be considered less of a headache if employers hire non-disabled people. Less expensive means the more attractive option.

Then there's difficulty of accessing services which can put a strain on our mental health. I can wholeheartedly attest to this. It is something that is significantly overlooked, but something that definitely needs to be resolved.

"In 2022, a report by the Welsh Parliament's Health and Social Care Committee concluded that not only do these groups [disability] have the most difficulty in accessing services, even when they do get support, their experiences and outcomes are poorer. It suggests the inequalities are deep-rooted within our society and it, therefore, requires a great deal of focus and radical thinking to overcome." – [Lesley Griffiths, Member of the Senedd for Wrexham]

The waiting times to see a social worker, gain access to physiotherapy services, hydrotherapy services, and even necessary equipment is shameful. You need support from these services if you have a disability to feel some kind of independence and benefit. When you do eventually get in the system, and are seen, you can guarantee that the service you're receiving won't last forever. Why? Money. Money rules everything, and unfortunately this includes disability. Realistically, to resolve this, Government needs to prioritize disability in the budget. Then, I can guarantee that Lesley Griffiths' quote would be irrelevant.

Inaccessibility, ableism, patronisation, social denial, ignorance, manipulation, judgement, vulnerability, and assumptions are just some things a person with a disability faces every single day. Adding a mental health issue into this battle, making people aware of the mental health issue isn't an attractive prospect. Staying silent is. We have enough to deal with as it is in terms of ableism, without the added stress of extra labels being thrust upon us. We are arguably seen as vulnerable as it is, without giving society more ammunition to double down on this belief.

Disrespecting Disability with Death

Recently, (as of writing this), I spoke to one of my colleagues from the *Ling Trust*, Jayne Knight, and she brought up the topic of general society blatantly disrespecting people who have a disability of some form, when a person in general either has a debilitating illness, and/or at the end of their life.

Factors

It is widely said that people in general society blatantly say, (and I'm paraphrasing):

"If ever I become ill, or develop a disability of some form, please just kill me."

Self-respect can be used as a reason as to why a person may say this. If you reach this stage in your life where you may become more dependent on others, if you have lived independently throughout your life, I can imagine the prospect of having to rely on others maybe a jarring notion. Having that choice of assisted suicide maybe considered a 'better alternative'. As a society, anything that can potentially jeopardise our independence and dignity is often seen as a big no-no. Having the choice to end your life if it has indeed panned out this way maybe an attractive prospect and/or solution.

Who are you hurting, and possibly offending though if you believe this?

A person with a disability.

There was a recent programme on TV from British actress, comedian, broadcaster and disability rights activist, Liz Carr.

Better Off Dead was a documentary presented by Liz Carr on assisted suicide. The subject matter is a real important topic to cover. Disability is ultimately seen as a negativity. I remember being told in secondary school, *"why can't you just die? You're a waste of a life anyway."* Obviously, the negative impact not only this, but similar comments had on my mental well-being was a lot to say the least.

Going back to look at how society perceives disabilities, ultimately saying, (and in most cases, very matter of fact), the desire or just the attraction of having the option to end a life over something as insignificant as developing a disability of some form (especially if that disability is only physical), can be a really difficult thing for those with disabilities to hear. You are really just banding us together into one group. There's no chance for individuality. To society, a disability means inability. Once a person has reached this stage in life, then it's seen as the end anyway. For those living with disabilities, this

Factors

type of language is discriminate, ableist, degrading, stereotyping and isolating all rolled into one. How do you think hearing this makes us feel? We are just bottom of the food chain, we're pathetic, unable to do things, dependant, a burden to society, a fate worse than death, quite literally. It's abhorrent behaviour. If you're in constant discomfort and unable to do tasks however, this is a very different outlook. I was just talking about those in society who have cognitive abilities but still chooses to say discriminating things just because they may not like the idea of a **possibility** of becoming disabled, having to rely on others. I get it, independence and dignity are important, but by disrespecting disability, society themselves are ultimately taking **our** independence and dignity away.

In a society where disabled people are often told they are 'better off dead' than disabled, Liz asks:

"Should we really be giving more power to end that group of people's lives?" – [Liz Carr, Actress, comedian, broadcaster and disability rights activist]

240

The thing is, I feel anyway, because we are seen as vulnerable, (treated like children), our own cognitive abilities get ignored, because people are just focused on what they may see, or even may misunderstand about the subject, disregarding the **human being**, opting seamlessly to concentrate on the disability. This is what's important, (I fee at least), to society, physicality and/or unintelligence. Things that can welcome unwanted actions like manipulation and/or sympathy. Again, I assume people behave like this towards those people who have a disability because they may not know how else to react, and so the automatic go to interaction is just to manipulate, sympathise, empathise and patronise because it's what society's been exposed to for centuries it seems. We're seen as unintelligent and vulnerable, so people can find it easy to interact with a person who has a disability of some form, because of this reasoning, because society believes a false narrative over reality.

Assisted Dying Bill

At the end of November 2024, UK Government will vote on a bill which will affect assisted dying.

Factors

Currently there's a lot of backlash and controversy on the topic, unsurprisingly from the current Health Minister Wes Streeting and other MPs, alongside Baroness Tanni Grey-Thompson DBE. If the bill is passed, then it will give people the choice of dying if they develop an illness which will have a negative impact on life. Apparently, there is proper safeguarding in this particular bill which will hopefully stop any abuse to the system.

In all honesty, currently I'm on the fence. Both arguments can have serious consequences to mental health. I understand all arguments for and against the bill. To support the bill, I can completely understand the mental anguish denial of choice can cause if a person is suffering significantly, especially with a terminal illness, but I also understand the apprehension it could cause if the bill is passed in terms of potential misuse, and mental health implications which of course, is a worrying prospect. Baroness Grey-Thompson DBE has said she will vote against the bill, simply because of how people with disabilities are treated, concurring with myself actually that if you have a disability, you don't have a choice in life. If the bill is passed, it can have serious consequences with those who have a disability deciding to end their life, as it's the only choice they would have. This in itself is a really sobering thought.

UK Government has apparently undertaken extensive research, looking at how other country's safeguarding is implemented, and hopes to learn lessons from that safeguarding approach other countries have adopted, but improving the safety by conditioning it.

Baroness Grey-Thompson DBE has said that even though safeguarding will be in place, there's no guarantee that the safeguarding will last.

Safeguarding anything that can pose potential danger and misuse to the public is the responsible thing to do. It's crucial. Maintaining that safeguarding is essential. Over time, there's a risk of safeguarding diminishing due to human error and/ or ignorance. Dreams work. Ideas work, but if you aren't willing to put in the work to execute those ideas and dreams, well, what's the point? There will

Factors

come a time when monitoring safeguarding becomes less of an issue, opening society up to fail, therefore, keeping issues with our mental health alive, and more worryingly, the prospect of death either by self-infliction or at the hands of others.

If you're terminally ill and in constant pain, then this bill could be the thing that appeals to you. Existence isn't living, and sadly if you are at this stage where you're feeling that you are just existing rather than living due to a terminal illness and assisted dying is an option, knowing that you have that option maybe comforting, not only to you, but others around you. Andrew Ranger MP for Wrexham is voting for the bill as he has apparently heard from people in society who have shared their own personal stories (of which I've decided not going to divulge due to privacy and respect, but I wanted to mention it to show the different factors that are dividing the nation at the moment.

I really don't have an answer on this as both points are valid in my opinion. I guess we will just have to see what transpires.

29.11.2024 Update:

The UK Government has today passed the 1st stage of the bill for making assisted dying legal. As you can imagine there's continued controversy. I'm personally worried for how this law will impact people with disabilities after really thinking about it. We're seen as unintelligent and vulnerable, and this assumption may impact on how assisted dying is used. Yes, there may be safeguarding, but how is that safeguarding being monitored? Will it continue to be monitored in years to come? How safe will people with disabilities be? I truly understand the want for those with a terminal illness, but is there a clause in the bill excluding people with disabilities if they aren't terminally ill? How safe is the safeguarding? There is also a real danger of internalised ableism here, as people with disabilities may feel like they're a burden to loved ones, and so may believe that the bill is an ideal 'solution' to end the struggle and stress for others.

This bill shouldn't be used as a means to ease the burden on others, or make others feel burdensome to the point of believing that ending life is the answer. Personally I fear as the years go on; this is exactly what will happen. I'm not trying to fear monger, I'm just being realistic.

There's still a long way to go before the bill is fully passed, but as it currently stands, the bill is looking likely to become law. This will only work if the safeguarding is continuous. There cannot be any lapses in any way. I just fear that this will be misused regardless of the safeguarding in place. I'm just really fearful now for the future.

Social Intrusion

Asking intrusive questions is another example of disrespecting people who have disabilities.

"I usually assume invasive questions, or asking if I tried everything,...I think it is because they believe I did something to deserve a disability, then, because they think they are good people, they can't get a horrible disease or have a terrible accident and become disabled..." – ['Jme' Elias, social media participant]

Expecting the invasive questions says a lot about the relationship between society, disability and mental health. There obviously isn't a relationship. Thinking that disabilities only happen to others in society is a naivety which is completely comical to me. People with disabilities are usually deemed naive, however, society is, in fact themselves, naive for misinterpreting the reality of disability.

In reality, anyone can become disabled at any point in their lives. Nobody is immune or has superpowers to 'fix' themselves if an illness or develops a disease which may affect their mobility or cognitive abilities.

People, I really do think, doesn't understand (or chooses to ignore) how intrusive questions may negatively impact on mental health. Asking intrusive questions only cements the false narrative that disability is equal to difference. Why should disability be intriguing? It really isn't anyone's concern other than the person with a disability themselves. How will asking extremely personal, (and by in large, humiliating) questions to another person in society who is deemed 'vulnerable'

Factors

anyway, enhance your life? What do you stand to gain? It makes no logical sense whatsoever. It makes me angry that society feels like they have a right to ask personal questions, that really isn't anyone's concern except for the person with the disability, unless you truly want to learn without any ulterior motives. However, I highly doubt that by asking intrusive questions, society will learn the truth about disability. I fail to see why anyone would ask questions that are personal and unnecessary. Yes, I could be considered sceptical for not trusting society's intensions, but we do live in a *Big Brother* type of world today where everything is less private and under surveillance more. Case in point, a lot of participants said that they have faced questions about intimacy, just to give one example of confusing interactions. Why is this beneficial for people to know? How would this information be beneficial to others in society? It's just inconceivable and outrageous to have such questions asked. General society never have these types of questions bombard them, so why does a person with a disability have to deal with these abhorrent questions? It's one rule for one, another rule for another. This behaviour will not improve the relationship between disability and mental health at all, it will only create further distance, segregation between the two demographics. Asking intrusive questions will only create more false assumptions about disability. Asking these types of questions really only confirms society's misunderstanding and stereotyping.

I've written about this before, but we as a human race, have 'main character syndrome'. We are the main character in our lives, and nobody else really matters, only ourselves. We may care for our family and friends, but we ultimately care about our own personal achievements, and how we are going to succeed in life, which is completely understandable to a point. The issue I have is when this behaviour negatively impacts on others in society. Climbing the societal hierarchy is good, everyone should strive to be the best they can, but not when this has a negative impact on others around them. It's just cruel to just blatantly ignore others, especially

Factors

those you may deem insignificant. This is when selfishness can rear its ugly head.

However, there are those individuals who may see someone they deem is useful to them, and is 'vulnerable', they can develop an arguably unhealthy obsessive fascination with their target. If these people believe that a person will have a profound impact on their lives (**not** in a positive way – only a belief that they can exploit this person that they have set their sights on for their own personal gains). These types of people may do everything in their power to gain the person's trust to make it easier to ultimately get what they want. As a result, manipulation maybe used to gain that trust. This is unfortunately what happened to me.

Experiencing this was an horrendous time period, not only affecting myself, but also regrettably, my family. I became a shadow of my former self. I was irritable, quiet, anxious and depressed. The manipulators promised me the world but delivered next to nothing. When I first met the manipulators, I wasn't in a good headspace, and they saw the opportunity to take full advantage. They played with my feelings, and my emotions. I tried to give them the benefit of the doubt for some unknown reason. I guess that I didn't want to believe that it was happening. I tried my very best to ignore what was happening and hide my mental health decline from the people responsible for creating this unrest in my mind. It was a real turbulent time in my life. I felt I needed to keep these people happy, by any means necessary, neglecting both myself and the most important people in my life, my own family. The deterioration of my mental health was quick. I'm not ashamed to admit that I was brainwashed. Nothing else mattered besides these people. They mistreated me, but I couldn't see it. I saw them through rose-tinted glasses, it was myself and everyone else who were wrong. It's so awful what manipulation can do, if your state of mind is low.

The Role of The Manipulator

Manipulators look for the weakest person in society, usually, manipulators opt for people who are considered vulnerable or emotionally exhausted. The person who often has low self-esteem. This is the preferred person, someone with no self-respect and who is considered dependent. They work hard to get you to trust them, for you to believe **everything** they say, arguably to an obsessive degree. They will often promise you the Earth. Why? I feel they do this to have a sense of power over others, to make themselves feel important. It's a type of control which they are more than happy to oblige to.

Manipulators tend not to deliver on what they promised you, making you feel that it's your fault as to why they haven't carried out the promise. Then, if you question the mistreatment, the manipulators often make you feel you have done something wrong by flagging the mistreatment up. As if you are overthinking the situation. They do this by praising you, by apologising, by replacing the original promise with another one, whatever they can do to try and make you feel guilty for calling into question the mistreatment. This is an attempt to try and cover themselves, save you exposing them and the truth. It's a never-ending cycle of narcissistic abuse. The truth is, manipulators will never keep to their promises, but they strategically know how to keep you on side, by constantly gas lighting you until you are hanging on their every word. You don't want to upset them, as you may lose them. Manipulators know this, and they take advantage. I don't need to do research on this as I know first-hand what happens, as it's happened to me. You may be asking why doesn't the person just leave the situation? The thing is, if you suffer from mental health issues anyway as a result of trauma, rejection, whatever, you are going to try and cling to the person or people who are showing you a crumb of attention, as you, (at the time), may believe it's genuine attention. Your judgement of the situation is clouded. This is how manipulators operate, by finding the weakest person they can, and exploiting them in a carefully orchestrated way for own their personal gains. Manipulators don't care how the mistreatment may affect their target. It's all about them, with the pretence of making you believe that they care for you and will do everything in their power to keep you happy. The reality is extremely different, however. Yes,

Factors

manipulators make sure that you are happy, but this checking in isn't selfless, it's selfish.

Disability is associated with vulnerability, so manipulators prefer people considered more vulnerable than others for obvious reasons. My own experience with manipulation had me question my own response to my manipulator's empty promises. I used to worry whether the reason why the promises never came to fruition was because I wasn't enthusiastic enough. The worry consumed me to the point where I felt it was **my duty** to make sure that I was more enthusiastic next time. Of course, this was pointless because no promises came, which of course made the worry worse.

Personal (Internalised Ableism)

Then finally, there's the personal implications of disability, also known as internalised ableism. There's an argument to be made that this personal implications/internalised ableism can be a response to environmental and/or societal challenges, but this isn't black and white.

Personal hate and self-loathing can develop at a young age. You may want to do things, you see others in society doing things, but you can't because you simply aren't as able. You may feel like a burden to those who are caring for you. Being dependent on others can be a serious issue for some with a disability, (especially when a person becomes disabled in later life).

Feelings of self-hatred can become continuous. These feelings can take root in your mind and not leave unless you get help in some way. This happened to me. I became vicious with myself and those around me. I absolutely despised myself. I started to believe everything that was thrown at me for so many years, add on top the blatant manipulation I was unfortunately experiencing at the time. I just became this unhappy, violent person. Regrettably now, I somehow believed that every single negative experience I had up to that point was due to me, and me alone. It must be, as it can't be everyone else in society who is wrong. I must be wrong. This was the conclusion I came to. After coming to this conclusion, I just gave up, I

Factors

surrendered to my disability. That's who I was at that point to the general public anyway, so I may as well embrace it. There was no use trying to fight it, people had already made up their minds anyway. This was the darkest period of my life. Giving up on yourself is a devastating thing to do. We have no opportunities, we are confined to our disabilities, we have no freedom. We are oppressed. Coming to terms with this is upsetting. For me, it was the acceptance that was the saddest thing of all. I worked so hard, but for what? I was a liability.

Sadly, this is the general consensus from people with disabilities to become despondent with themselves. We become a slave to the disability narrative. We become willing to play the part. Internalised ableism is a serious issue. It's self-sabotage.

Going back to Ben Ashby's comment, ignorance of a person with a disability can make you feel insecure and belittled. There's every chance of developing a mentality of giving up trying to participate in society because nobody gives you the chance to. Ignorance makes us feel worthless. I unfortunately, have experienced the same as Ben. It became apparent that people in society weren't going to take me seriously when colleagues in my 1st job, after graduating from university, preferred, and/or opted to speak to the support worker who was with me rather than speaking to me. The annoying thing was, the colleagues were asking my support worker at the time, work related things. The support worker didn't work for the company, I did. By deliberately ignoring me, it caused me really to spiral and question my own self-worth. My own self-esteem deteriorated significantly. It made me realise how my disability was going to be an issue for people and this realisation did give me food for thought on my own life, and who I actually was.

Why general society think that disability is also equal to unintelligence, is beyond me. There's no logical reason in the 21st century why this is accepted. There should be a lot more knowledge about disability today. We should have become more aware of the reality of disability, but sadly, we haven't. A disability doesn't always mean inability.

Factors

With this negative belief though, a person with a disability can feel trapped in the fake narrative of what disability means, rather than what it actually means. This feeling of entrapment can have knock on effects on those who are the target of the entrapment. Comparison can be a serious issue for those with disabilities.

Comparison

"Comparison is an act of violence against the self." – [Iyanla Vanzant, American inspirational speaker and lawyer]

Not a truer word spoken.

Comparison is the way of the world nowadays. We have an unhealthy obsession with comparing ourselves with others. The world is under surveillance 24/7 it seems, and our emotions are heightened. We have become a sensitive society. The world is more open to comparison and indeed, intrusion.

"...constantly comparing we to others can lead to feelings of inadequacy, jealousy, and low self-

esteem. We might start questioning our own abilities, thinking we're not good enough because we don't match up to someone else's achievements or lifestyle." – ['Why comparison affects your mental health', Published: 18 Feb 2024, Let's Talk About Mental Health]

These feelings of inadequacy, jealousy and low self-esteem are all feelings that a person with a disability can develop. Seeing others walk, do things easily, and just generally live a 'proper life'. These feelings of inadequacy and jealousy can lead to destructive behaviour patterns.

- Body image issues

- Self-harm

- Suicidal thoughts

These are extreme examples yes, but equally valid ones. There's no telling how ableism will affect a person. Everyone in life deals with things differently. Some maybe strong enough to let it wash over them, others however, may not be as emotionally resilient. These are the exact people who tend to get the brunt of the ableism. The quiet ones. Being quiet plays into the stereotype of disability – the vulnerability. The thing is, being silent maybe an adoptive tactic. Much like a defeatist attitude. People who are quiet may not actually be this way, it could be for the simple fact that others have made them this way through sheer ableism, inside though can be that once confident, self-assured person but they're buried under the hatred. Take it from me, it can be difficult to emerge from the hate unscathed if it has been constantly building over the years.

Personally, I never had any issues with seeing others living a life, by disability standards as a child, it was only later in life where this comparison issue took hold, when my disability became more apparent to society.

only a fleeting thought, but nothing that would ever significantly affect my mental health. I'm quite 'ordinary' (for want of a better word), I 'defy' what it means to have a disability in the eyes of society. I'm capable to live a relatively independent lifestyle. Of course, there are instances where I may need assistance, but really that's only personal care. I don't define myself as disabled. A very good friend of mine defined it perfectly, you're disabled by society. An extremely accurate description. Society disables you instantly by using that label, you may not define yourself as 'disabled', but society definitely does. I didn't realise how true this statement is, until I became an adult. There are those people who develop a mental health issue because society doesn't accept you. They only see one thing, a disability, and nothing more. For me personally, I'm okay with who I am. Would I like to have the opportunity to walk? In some respects, of course I would. When I was a child, I remember saying to mum on occasion that, "I wish I could walk", why I believe I said this was because seeing my friends on the playground or in the neighbourhood, running around, having fun, I guess I wished for that just to see what it was like to be able to properly use my legs without my wheelchair. I know that I wasn't jealous per say, because my friends always included me no matter what. I just wanted to see what it was like to

Factors

actually run. A simple thing, but an honest thing. This want though, never actually impacted on me mentally, it was a passing thought as a child, I did wonder what walking and running would be like, but this curiosity didn't impact on my mental health as a young child somehow. It did impact me when I started secondary school, but this was solely because of the mistreatment I faced daily in that environment.

As I've grown, I've realised and I've accepted (especially in recent years – since becoming an author really) that this is the hand I've been dealt, and I'm okay with it. I'm happy to be me. I'm back to how I used to be. As you may know by now, this feeling of happiness and contentment was a long time coming.

I've adapted to society, yet society hasn't adapted to me. Constantly being rejected over something that I cannot control daily, will ultimately lead to increased feelings of stress and anxiety for anyone, regardless of who you are. Accessibility, or indeed, lack of accessibility, is another reason why a disabled person's mental health may deteriorate. If inaccessibility occurs, this is only confirming the existence of ableism. Being denied access to anywhere is ultimately being denied access to life, I know that sounds dramatic, but it's true. People who have a disability of some form, often find it difficult to be as independent as they could've, simply because of the lack of accessibility in the world. Obviously, this can potentially cause mental health issues. I do wonder how would general society cope when faced with the lack of accessibility issue if they themselves were the main demographic who relied on a full accessible world? In short, society wouldn't. There undoubtedly would be absolute uproar if public places weren't accessible. People who have a disability, are treated as second class citizens, compared to the rest of the population, and the accessibility issue is partly why. The general public seems to be catered to mostly. We are an afterthought it seems.

"Accessibility limitations and challenges are frustrating. Being subject to these physical barriers on a daily basis can lead to mental wellness issues such as: Feelings of isolation and

Factors

abandonment." – ['What a Poor Accessibility Negatively Affects Your Mental Health', Home2Stay.com]

I know that I personally struggled with my mild Cerebral Palsy for many years in later life. I personally knew my capabilities, but making others see your capabilities if you have a disability is sadly an uphill and unnecessary battle. Trying to make people aware of your declining mental state, on top of what people often think of you, is simply too much. It's excessive.

The reason why I personally chose to keep quiet about my mental health issues were a combination of reasons. With a disability, it doesn't matter what kind, society often sees you as 'vulnerable' without seeing you as a person. You're effectively an object, without the extra label of issues with mental health. You are labelled as it is, we objectify disability, without anything else that's considered negative added to your 'personality', your sense of being. I didn't want that for myself understandably.

The other reason is that people may not understand or acknowledge your fragile mental state alongside having a disability of some form. I just felt that if I attempted to speak up about my ongoing mental decline, I would be segregated further. This is something that I definitely didn't want to potentially deal with, on top of everything I had to try to manage.

Somehow people are unable to understand that a disabled person may also have a mental health issue of some kind. I don't know why this is, but this is how the majority of society operates, not everyone in society admittedly, but the vast majority.

Chapter 10
"Congratulations! You can do things! You're amazing"

Often, this chapter's title is what it feels like when any person with a disability 'defies the odds. Condescending attitudes. It doesn't matter your disability, and even the severity of our disabilities, if we attempt to do something 'out of the ordinary' for a 'disabled person', something that is generally reserved for mainstream society, like obtaining qualifications, have a family, (or more rare), getting a good job, or even just hold a conversation, it's mundane, but it's treated as this marvellous thing when disability is added into that mix. I've had people patronise me even when they've learned about my educational background and my career. I've found that it goes either one way or another, either person immediately change their opinion of you, you go from 'vulnerable', to equal at a drop of a hat, (however, this is extremely rare). Or, strangely, (and I've had this, so I know), people can double

Congratulations!

down on their patronisation by saying things like *"aren't you clever?!"*

Ian Jarvis' experience sadly is common, but like I've said, it must be more difficult to accept this new existence if you've become a person with a disability later in life. You are now on the receiving end of the ableism. The mental anguish this may cause must be awful to say the least. To reiterate, Ian said:

"...if I'm on my own I suddenly seem interesting as though it's a surprise that I function very well on a mental level. For me this was really hard to come to terms with because I've always been independent so to suddenly be treated as less than a full person really knocked my confidence."
– [Ian Jarvis, social media participant]

Lack of confidence I would say, is one of the main feelings when it comes to disability. It is always seen that we aren't a 'full person', and it's a 'shame' that we have a disability of some kind. How do you think that type of language affects us? Are we going to agree with you? Are we going to play up to the fact?

If you become disabled later in life, I can imagine that this can be a jarring experience all round. Not only do you have to come to terms with your new way of life and adapt to it the best you can, but you also have to contend with the sympathetic looks, and newly found patronisation.

If we do things that aren't identified with disability, we are often described as 'inspirational'.

Why does this attitude still exist today? Why do we have to accept these types of patronising words as compliments? Tell me, why are we 'inspirational'? What makes us 'inspirational'? Just because we may succeed in something which others in general society find mundane? It's passive aggressive behaviour. It may seem as if you are encouraging, but ultimately you are silently saying that *"you are amazing for what you've achieved **despite your disability**."* As if our disabilities are an automatic blocking mechanism. Even if you don't realise you are being patronising, the hidden meaning in your

Congratulations!

words is clear to us. You, yourself is the automatic blocking mechanism. By saying things like this, you are just reminding us that we are connected to disability. We cannot be anything more. We are destined to be 'disabled' and nothing else. Our achievements don't have any bearing. Our achievements don't take precedence over disability. Your words only remind us that it doesn't matter what we do, we will always be weighted down. You are only buying into the stereotype. It makes us feel insecure and belittled. The mental health implications of your words and actions can be a distressing time.

I think I've spoken about this before, but there was one incident which happened to me where this blatant discrimination occurred. I was at a family party, and someone came up to me (someone who I didn't know that well, and subsequently didn't know me that well), and said that it was a shame that I was disabled. This made me angry, but I calmly and assertively listed all of my achievements. I remember saying *"Well, it's* okay, because I graduated from university with a BSc Honours degree in graphic design, and I'm a freelance graphic designer for the motorsport industry, so I've done quite well for myself considering." Usually, I don't like to list everything that I've done for fear of sounding like I'm better than everyone else, which of course I'm not. Yes, I've worked hard, but I don't like to announce it to the world by rule, but you feel like you have to if you have a disability of some form, in order to try and educate people around you. This is what makes me uncomfortable. Others don't have to explain their achievements. It just really infuriates me that I have to just because I'm in a wheelchair. I was with my sister-in-law Ceri at the time of that incident, and she said the look of complete shock on this person's face when we moved away was incredible. This person didn't expect me to be as coherent, successful and independent as I was. They were expecting the stereotype. I just said to Ceri that it needed to be done. I don't like doing it, but people leave me no choice.

Higher education is hard work for everyone, regardless of who you are. It's non-stop. The

Congratulations!

constant pressure is immense. Often, you stay up all night to get one assignment done before a deadline, only for another assignment to immediately crop up. Why would anyone put themselves through that? Ultimately, for a better life, with the promise of a good job at the end of the blood, sweat and tears. That's meant to be your reward. After all, you deserve it. You've earned it. However, this isn't the reality for general society, nevertheless those who have a disability of some form. A person with a disability has less chance of obtaining and keeping a good job, or even a job at all. All that we get are rejections, and also places that claim to be for people with disabilities, undermining you by pandering to the disability instead of talking to you as an equal. Often, we are spoken to slowly and softly. This is demeaning. This attitude instantly makes us feel different. Most of the time, these places (or groups) have speakers come in with worksheets and ask you to do very basic, very simple tasks, regardless of who you actually are. This is what I mean when I say that society just see one element of you, not the whole of you, (even though society claims to), it's just sad.

You would think that we've just attempted to fly over the Atlantic – something extraordinary - judging by the extreme amount of wonderment and patronisation that is shown. When people in general society are confronted with this 'ordinary, and mundane lifestyle', nobody bats an eye. Compare this to a person with a disability achieving exactly the same goals, well, that's just incredible and fascinating. Why should there be a hidden barrier? How does this work? How is Government allowing such prejudice and ableism? Can it work long-term? This in itself is extremely dangerous on one's mental health. Congratulating us on a "job well done" if we so much as ever do anything that goes against what is understood to have a disability is demeaning. Basically, we just want the opportunity to be able to showcase our abilities. Always being denied an everyday life over something as insignificant as a disability is immoral, it would get you in the end, that mental health decline. We are just expected to comply to the

Congratulations!

forced narrative of disability, stay silent, and be okay about it. This **isn't** a democracy, only a dictatorship. This description may sound harsh without context, but you try living with a disability of some form. I can guarantee you will ultimately feel **exactly** the same as I do currently.

We are actually equal to the non-disabled people in society, in reference to how the constant mistreatment will ultimately lead to mental health decline. The non-disabled arguably are better treated than those who are considered disabled.

If a non-disabled person loses employment because of a ridiculous reason, or if a non-disabled person cannot gain access to a building simply because of an easily resolved issue, and nothing is done to rectify the situation, or whatever it is, you can guarantee that changes would definitely be made, as there would be uproar if nothing was done.

The uproar concern is certainly dampened down if you have a disability. People always automatically place those negative prefixes onto you if you mention disability in any context. We are 'vulnerable', 'naive', 'weak', just every single negative description, we unfortunately have to conform to, accept and shut up.

I talked about ableism, (obviously in my last book, *Disabling Ableism),* which basically is like a form of discrimination that is solely aimed towards disability, and **nothing** screams ableism more than this obvious barrier that society creates.

Why should we be congratulated on living a life? Congratulating us on things that others in society are allowed to do easily without fuss, only reinforces those negative stereotypes of disability. You may think that you are being kind and caring by saying well done for something as simple as ordering a meal in a restaurant for example, but in actuality, you are only reinforcing the negative stereotypes that disability is recognised for. This instantly makes us feel different to others in society. This makes us feel like we aren't equal to the rest of the world, almost as if we are helpless new-born babies, or even aliens. This ultimately will only encourage mental health issues.

Congratulations!

Throughout all of this negative reinforcement, we are just expected to stay silent in the face of adversity, and just accept our place in society, the bottom of the food chain, the bottom of social hierarchy. No. Why should we? We aren't respected for **us**. We aren't respected **at all**. This would play on anyone's mental health deterioration regardless of who you are, wouldn't it if you're constantly under surveillance 24/7 and congratulated for something as simple as putting a cup away in a cupboard? I know this example is extreme, but I argue that people's reactions to us doing simple, mundane tasks is equally, if not more extreme.

Chapter 11
The Rise of Social Media = The Rise of Ableism?

As already alluded to in this book, society has become increasingly obsessed with social media and by extension, media in general. Privacy isn't well respected today. Everyone has access to everything. Our lives aren't our own. We live in a world run by media and social media. Everything is examined under a microscope. Our whole life is portrayed online, which lends itself to mental health decline.

People with disabilities seem to be more open to abuse and exploitation online, probably because of the anonymity aspect of it. It's more appealing to abuse, cyber-bully and exploit when you're anonymous. It's a step removed. As the instigator, you can distance yourself from the situation. It's awful and unethical, but sadly true.

There's a perfect example of disability abuse further in this chapter. I do believe that it's because of the

The Rise of Ableism?

lack of education around the subject. Again, the education subject is mentioned, but this will be covered in more detail in the next chapter, but because of this lack of education, people with disabilities tend to often be the target of online abuse and cyber-bullying, because we are seen as vulnerable and an easy target which isn't based in reality. It's just a stereotypical viewpoint. A viewpoint which is outdated and offensive in many ways

This belief is based on appearance and assumptions of the past.

Ableism isn't just isolated to abuse either, ableism can be due to lack of accessibility and unfortunately, in this day and age too, this type of ableism can extend to social media. Why this is, I feel is due to cost. Money runs the world and sadly this can mean potential accessibility issues. Accessibility is a human right and cost should never be an issue. Why should cost prevent people with disabilities from having access to things others do? It's discrimination. As I keep saying, we are segregated and isolated as it is due to public perceptions. Comparing ourselves constantly with general society, thus creating the internalised ableism we can sadly experience as a result.

We shouldn't be denied access to the online world just because of lack of funding. The inaccessibility factor only plays into the stereotype, thus creating more animosity between disability and general society, thus creating or sustaining mental health issues for those with disabilities.

For people with disabilities, lack of funding goes hand in hand with disability unfortunately, we cannot obtain the equipment we need to live as independently as possible, we cannot access ongoing activities such as hydrotherapy due to lack of funding. Now social media is affected by making accessibility a luxury, and so, is unaffordable? There shouldn't be a price on accessibility. Accessibility is a basic human right. How do you think it makes us feel when something as simple as technology should at least be fully accessible. It's technology after all, but it isn't accessible to people with disabilities at all. This is an oxymoron. It's ridiculous. No wonder people with disabilities are more susceptible to mental health decline. Wouldn't you be if you were denied to live constantly?

Pandemic

Now, this isn't to say that social media especially, doesn't have its benefits. Social media was originally designed and created to be a connector, especially those with disabilities ironically. A very humble and positive intention. This initial intention became more apparent during the COVID-19 pandemic. During the pandemic, we as a human race were segregated and isolated. It feels ironic to me that people with disabilities are often isolated and segregated anyway, it was quite interesting, to me at least, seeing how the whole world coped with this sudden change in everyday life. The answer was unsurprisingly, not that well in a physical sense at least. Mental health decline increased immensely during the pandemic. Government at the time didn't help matters as the information given was extremely contradictory and confusing. There was a real unknown during this period of time, hence the mental health decline increase. There was fear and uncertainty. However, for all of the anxiety inducing feelings the pandemic created, society actually became more resilient, more friendly, more together ironically thanks to social media of all things.

We weren't taking things for granted anymore. We started making the most of any small interaction we had. It was like an Armageddon type of mentality during this period of time, so society decided to come together online to socialise. Everyone was in the exact same situation, so there wasn't any superiority or ego to contend with. Arguably and ironically, the pandemic became a positive experience for the kindness of humanity. The pandemic showed how we can positively interact with each other without any toxicity. We became so grateful for any kind of interaction. We became a kinder world.

This new global determination to support each other should have remained, but unfortunately, I feel that as we have slowly returned to the world we knew without fear, we have forgotten the important things. People. Family, friends, acquaintances, we have just forgot to check in and

The Rise of Ableism?

spend quality time with one another. Our busy lives that were once dead during the pandemic, have been reborn and as a direct result, so has our ignorance. Arguably, we were more willing to talk to each other during the pandemic, and we were more concerned for those around us, especially people with disabilities and the elderly. We were willing and more importantly, wanting to communicate with these people in society, not having anything else happening, it will make you much more aware of your surroundings, and the people who live in those surroundings.

I just wish we hadn't lost that mentality, but as the saying goes:

"The world keeps turning."

I just wish that the world would keep turning with awareness, especially that awareness of those who have disabilities, and mental health issues. There needs to be acknowledgement of these two subjects being interlinked. Social media is a great place to start this revolution. It can be mined numbing and tedious to live the same invisible life day to day. Willingness to learn and change for the better regarding social attitudes and beliefs, because it isn't enough just to say the things, belief in what you are saying is crucial. If we don't have belief, there's absolutely no point in saying something. There needs to be power behind the words.

Social media became the go to for socialisation and togetherness. During this time, social media finally became the force for good, what it was originally created for. As said before, we are social creatures by nature, and when you couldn't physically socialise with others, (including your friends and loved ones), social media became the ideal solution. We, for a little while at least, became caring, kind, and friendly.

People with disabilities, (although not the main target demographic), found social media to be a huge part of finding friends to interact with. It can still be a positive for people with disabilities, especially those who cannot physically leave the house, or their disability prevents them from developing potential relationships in person, such

The Rise of Ableism?

as a person with a learning disability of some kind for example. Social media can be the perfect alternative for those who are unable to maintain physical relationships for one reason or another.

"People with physical and sensory and/or learning disabilities may find it more difficult to connect with people and generate or sustain new friendships. They may become socially isolated and lonely, which can have a serious impact on a person's health and emotional wellbeing." – ['Independent living: Friendships and relationships', Devon.org.uk]

So, in some ways, social media can be a really great alternative to physical contact if you feel that physical contact is too anxiety inducing for one reason or another.

The thing is though, if you have a disability, deformity or illness of some kind, unfortunately you can expect this good experience to be minimal, because this initial good intention has become tainted over time. We have ruined the initial concept of social media. Social media has become the biggest antagonist to society. Bullying has become even more prominent than ever before because of social media. There's a real problem today with how we interact with each other. People with disabilities do seem to get the brunt of the abuse.

"...sites like Facebook and Twitter have become breeding grounds for very real hate. New research by the disability charity Leonard Cheshire, released today, shows online disability hate crime has soared in the last year, with recorded incidents up by almost a third...One young woman with extensive facial scarring spoke of being repeatedly mocked in public, with children on local school buses banging on bus windows to get her attention as she goes by. Some passers-by took her photograph and posted it on social media; others then posted hateful comments about her and tagged her to ensure she saw the abuse" – ['Online abuse of disabled people is getting worse – when will it be taken seriously?', Dr. Francis Ryan, Published: Fri 10 May 2019, The Guardian]

The Rise of Ableism?

Why is this still a thing? Why is this allowed to happen? It's just horrific, and absolutely terrifying. Yes, I realise that the article is from 2019, but you cannot ignore the blatant ableism on display here with this one young woman, and sadly this isn't an isolated incident.

"Three in ten disabled people (29 per cent) have experienced bullying or trolling online. More than half (53 per cent) have seen negative comments about disabled people or disability in general. Younger people are the hardest hit group with almost half of 18- to 34-year-olds enduring negative comments online." – ['Scope reveals shocking levels of online trolling experienced by disabled people', Published: 1st August 2023, Scope]

If you have been bullied as a non-disabled person for whatever reason, you know how bad it makes you feel. Bullying knocks your confidence, it's intimidating, it makes you feel isolated, lonely, fearful, dreading what the next day may bring. Bullying just stops you from living. If you are bullied because of your appearance for example, you have the option to change it, of course, you shouldn't have to, but this is the world we live in today, when everything is run on image.

The image issue does become the main problem if you have a disability, deformity or illness of some kind, especially if it's physical. People generally find it easier to criticise something that they think is unusual, something that is out of the ordinary, something that goes against the grain of what 'normal' is. Something that can be seen. Visibility is the most important thing to identify something.

Disability is something that a person cannot control. You don't have a choice; you cannot just decide that you're not going to have your disability one day. Disability doesn't work like that. So, in actuality, if you are bullied if you have a disability of some form, can arguably be worse, because you can't do anything to stop it. I can tell you, that it's absolutely heart-breaking. You just feel useless, feeble, faulty, enemy no. 1, targeted constantly, labelled, hurt. You actually feel dead inside. You don't feel worthy of life.

The Rise of Ableism?

Obsession is another negative that has come to the forefront of social consciousness. Pressures to look, and/or act a certain way are heightened. Comparison is the biggest issue when it comes to social media and media in general. *"Why can't I look like them?" "Why can't my life be like theirs?" "They seem to have everything." "They are doing well in life, what am I doing?"* This does seem to be the general consensus when it comes to our online lives.

When I was in the midst of my mental health deterioration, I used to look on social media, and seeing friends who I used to go to primary school with, either getting married, getting a good job, or getting pregnant, made me question where my life was headed. I felt like a complete failure in comparison. Yes, I graduated from university, but that was about it for my achievements up to that point in time. In my mind, graduating was pointless, as no employer would give me the time of day, let alone employment once they found out about my mild Cerebral Palsy, and the employers who would employ me, would only manipulate me. This wasn't a good time in my life. I became resentful of everyone and their 'successes' on social media. Jealousy became my main emotion. Why should others have a life, which is arguably considered successful by social standards, when I can't even have the opportunity to have a job interview without unfounded preconceptions? It just felt unfair to learn that really, it's one rule for one, another rule for another. I was being punished it seemed over something that was out of my control. Seeing others doing well, when effectively, I wasn't? No wonder I began to resent myself and others around me. Lack of opportunities will do this to you.

People, as I've now discovered, only put a small percentage of their lives on social media, the good moments. The reality is often much more different. People only let you see what they want you to see. They have full control, full power, which arguably, is absolutely right. People deserve the right to have control over their own lives. It's empowering more than anything. Where I personally take issue is when this power becomes self-indulgent and

The Rise of Ableism?

negatively impacts on others. You aren't getting the full, true picture. It's a snapshot. A sugar-coat. There's a lot of false information put out on social media and media in general, which are designed to make the poster fall into the false narrative of the 'perfect life', and in turn, make the rest of us (the viewers of the post) question ourselves, question our abilities, question our physicality.

Social media can play a significant negative part in the lives of young people if they unknowingly let it. It's bad enough for non-disabled young people to contend with, as the bills, and money worries may keep piling up and you're constantly seeing others live this 'cushy and easy' life, as if it comes naturally. This cannot be easy to deal with anyway, let alone introducing a disability into the mix. A disability can make our lives a living hell with social attitudes, on top of the potential added stress of what a non-disabled person goes through. In no way am I comparing situations, pitting them against each other in order to find out which demographic has it worse. I would never do that, as it can possibly lead to further division and segregation. We need to start closing the gap on this disability Apartheid, not widen it further.

Images that have been airbrushed are just one main reason for feelings of insecurity. Social media has been allowed to manifest as a negative. I think it's because on social media, anyone can be whoever they want to be, there's no limitation, which out of context, can be considered a good thing, but this can also lend itself to becoming a person with no moral compass. You are able to hide behind an account, a screen. The sense of power this can create in people can be devastating. This new feeling of power and entitlement can have detrimental effects on others in society, especially those who already have low self-esteem.

People in society seem to be dependent on social media, our lives are run by technology. In a way, we have become robots, slaves to devices, and what's on those devices. Social media has the ability to either use its platform as a positive, by connecting with others, having meaningful conversations etc. This positivity though is miniscule compared to what is actually posted on social media websites.

The Rise of Ableism?

Hatred, discrimination, racism, homophobia, hate speech, and ableism are easier to execute behind a screen rather than face to face. It's a move which is deemed cowardice, but a move that happens all too often. For one example, and this example isn't connected to disability, but it's a real good example of how misinformation of any kind can have negative consequences on the general public.

What I'm alluding to are the recent riots in the summer of 2024. I'm not going to go into the reason for the riots, as this isn't my place, I have no permission nor want to discuss this in full. There's absolutely no need to. What I am going to say is those riots were a direct result of a devastating incident. People on social media became riled up so much after the incident happened. False information was circulating, and this false information then made society susceptible to believing what they read or heard, and then acting on their feelings with their actions causing even more damage and destruction.

I just wanted to mention the above as an example of how social media can be quick to spread misinformation. This misinformation can alsc be connected to disability. I know this, as when I've conducted research for my books, almost all the information is negative. According to the Internet, as a whole, if you have a disability of some form, you cannot do anything. This mentality can spill onto other outlets like social media.

Chapter 12
Society's Complicated Social Media Relationship

Yes this book subject is covering disability's relationship to mental health. This is the main topic. However, in order to fully understand ableism and social media, I feel it's crucial to look at general society's relationship with social media.

Why Have We Become So Obsessed with Social Media?

It's easier to become the person we want to be online, versus who we actually are in reality. Likes, followers, friends, comments and shares are all triggers, triggers that release the hormone dopamine in our brains, which gives us a sense of pleasure and satisfaction. As already mentioned, we can be anyone we want to be on social media, there's no limitations, which can be an attractive prospect for many, especially if we are considered bottom of the food chain so to speak in reality, in

A Complicated Relationship

social circles, i.e. disabled. We can create a fictitious life, the life we wish we had, the life we crave, but can never obtain for one reason or another.

This obsession with social media actually has a name:

Social media addiction

Knowing that this is a thing, a recognised issue is an issue in itself. What we crave is approval and popularity to satisfy our own skewed idea of what having a great life means. There was an obsession on a certain social media website years ago (which I'm not too sure if it still exists today), but you always tried to get as many 'friends' as possible in order to confirm your 'popularity'. It was absolutely horrifying, when reflecting back now, but this just exemplifies the obsessive tendencies I'm talking about.

You see, social media is fake, 'friends' on social media are fake as they are only avatars. 'Likes' aren't real. Everything on social media is how we would like our lives to be, but in doing so, we are increasingly losing ourselves as a person in the process. Hence the slave comment earlier. This obsession to obtain as many 'likes' and 'friends', can ironically make us feel isolated and lonely, especially if we are cyber-bullied, don't get the amount of 'likes' we thought we were going to get, (if we receive any at all). We can beccme disassociated with reality. Living for just our on'ine 'lives'. Craving constant approval and attention.

Becoming A Cyber-bully

Social media can also harbour those who live to cause distress to others. Again, as already said, social media is an attractive place for cyber-bullying, ableism, hate speech, discrimination and other negatives. It's arguably the perfect place to act on negativity as you have the ability to remain anonymous on social media.

Bullying VS. Cyber-bullying: Which Is More Tolerable?

Bullying in any sense isn't tolerable, this question is redundant. It doesn't matter how, at the end of the

A Complicated Relationship

day, bullying is bullying. It can be relentless, intense and can affect a person's mental health.

However, years ago, (and arguably), it was easier if you were unfortunately the target for standard bullying for some reason. (For this section, I will refer to face to face bullying as standard bullying, in order to differentiate between the 2 terms, in order to save any confusion). In the past, if you were bullied in school, work, or in your neighbourhood, yes it may have been physical, emotional, verbal, or all of the above, but at least you only had to deal with it at certain times of the day. You had the option to have respite from the standard bullying by shutting your bully/bullies out at the end of the day, by physically shutting the door on it. You did have your own mind to contend with when the bullying stopped, and the worry that could consume you, but there was more of a chance of someone stepping in to stop the bullying.

Cyber-bullying is a whole other story.

A Complicated Relationship

Cyber-bullying has no off switch, it's constant, 24/7, and terrifyingly can go under the radar anonymously where nobody can intervene.

Everyone has access to social media, and as a direct result, everyone has access to each other's lives. With the option to remain anonymous, there's also the added worry of not knowing who is antagonising you. It may give people more incentive to bully others in a way, as there is a high chance of no ramifications. It can give a potential cyber-bully a sense of power.

Disability cyber-bullying is more appealing to a bully. We are seen as 'easy targets', willing to believe everything someone says. I do believe that it's how disability is perceived in society as to why people come to that conclusion.

People with learning disabilities statistically are more likely to be the target for cyber-bullying.

"Adults with learning disabilities may be more at risk of cyber bullying. This could be because they are more trusting, unaware to the fact that they are being bullied, or simply because seen as easy

targets to torment." – ['What Is Cyber-bullying?', Anncrafttrust.org]

I really do not trust statistics, as they could be manipulated to feed this notion that disability is equal to vulnerability, and vulnerability is equal to cyber-bullying, but it should be noted that people with learning disabilities are more trusting,

So, Why Do People Feel the Need to Bully?

People can become a bully for so many reasons. This isn't to say that these reasons are acceptable, because there's absolutely no justification to bully anyone, but some people react to situations differently and may think that becoming a bully is justified in their mind.

According to the Australian Government, some reasons are:

- *Wanting to dominate others and improve their social status.*

- *Having low self-esteem and wanting to feel better about themselves*

- *Having a lack of remorse or failing to recognise their behaviour as a problem*

- *Feeling angry, frustrated or jealous*

- *Struggling socially*

- *Being the victim of bullying themselves*

[Information from: Healthdirect.gov.au]

These reasons are devastating, and there's also a few more:

- Neglect

- Abuse

- Misunderstanding

- Disruptive home life

- Isolation

As I've mentioned before in my writing career, I'm not a psychologist, but to me, it is interesting that bullying others can be as a direct result of what is happening in your life, does say a lot about that person in my opinion. From my experience however, bullying is mostly due to jealousy, as

A Complicated Relationship

established, it's not the main reason by any means, as the above shows, but in my personal experience, jealousy does seem to be a main cause. Jealousy of the 'perfect life' that you may see or hear about, when your own life is basically 'non-existent' compared to what you're exposed to, especially online, so in order to regain control, bullying and cyber-bullying maybe an easier option to diminish other's self-esteem. It's so sad this is what people may resort to in order to feel a little better about themselves, by hurting others, either physically, emotionally or verbally, (admittedly, more emotional and verbal nowadays, given the way we live today), but unfortunately, this is where we are. This is the world today.

Chapter 13
The Education Debate

From my research for *Disabling Ableism*, the overall consensus when the topic of disability education came up, was the concern of teaching about disability, in schools especially, due to potential time constraints. My response to this valid concern was equally simple, teach about disability during periods of learning about society. I know for a fact that PSE (Personal Social Education), or PSHE (Personal Social Health Education) is still taught in secondary schools to this day, according to my sister-in-law Ceri, who's an English teacher in secondary school education. These sessions are perfect to educate about disabilities. When I had PSE lessons in secondary school, they taught about every aspect of life, managing money, CV writing, sex, bullying, puberty, contraception, pregnancy etc., which as mentioned before, are extremely effective and important topics to teach, however, disability, race, religion etc., was never touched. Probably because of the fear of offending, which is

The Education Debate

understandable, but this fear that society has, ultimately will only exasperate the issues further. In my own personal opinion (and I don't know how the reaction will be received once I say this by the way) but by actively **choosing** to ignore important topics such as disability, the education system is only encouraging further ableism and mental health deterioration in the long run. It isn't just my experience either, others with disabilities have experienced bullying in education.

"As a teenager I experienced bullying which led to my eating disorder and self-esteem issues..." – [Rachel Williams, social media participant]

This reason alone should be enough to turn the tide on disability education. It's no secret by now that I experienced bullying in secondary school due to my Cerebral Palsy, and it did affect me badly, as stated previously. Nobody should ever feel insignificant to anyone else in society. Yes, it's secondary school and so the stakes are much higher. Image, your personality, how you conduct yourself all play a part in your popularity status. That's the only thing that matters in secondary school, you're judged from your very first day, and that initial judgement stays with you throughout.

If being bullied because of your disability causes you to develop severe and dangerous issues later in life, then I feel that disability should be commonplace in education, period. There shouldn't be any apprehension. Eating disorders are serious, self-esteem issues are serious. These issues should **never** be swept under the carpet in the hope they will disappear. You cannot bury your head in the sand. It is the Education Department's responsibility to ensure that **every** aspect of life is taught. You cannot pick and choose. You can't in life, so you should **never** have the option to in education. The Education Department isn't doing a very good job at providing sensible, yet informative informaton when it is crucially needed. Education should be accessible to everyone, not just a certain part of the population, that's biased and discriminate. For people who have disabilities, it's ableist, pure and simple. Serious issues aren't a joke. You don't know what harm you maybe inflicting on a person with a disability. For Rachel, it was an eating disorder and issues with self-esteem, for me, it was a combination of self-harm, exponential dread, fear, isolation, loneliness, segregation, abuse, and depression. Being bullied over something that you cannot control is cruel and devastating. You do feel a deep feeling of all round resentment, not only for the person/people who feel like this, but also for yourself, (at least I did anyway.)

This is why I still believe that disability education is so important, which **should and needs** to be implemented throughout every part of school, from infants to university. In *Disabling Ableism*, this opinion was surprisingly controversial for many participants. It's the fear of the unknown I feel. Disability is still widely unknown by social standards. There are snippets of understanding, but these are only snippets. We need more knowledge about disability, and true knowledge, not common knowledge. Disability **deserves** more awareness, and not just this backhanded attempt. The backlash on this subject was immense in *Disabling Ableism*, society took issue with giving children extra work on top of everything else, and yes, I get it, of course I do. Extra unnecessary pressures can also cause mental health issues. However, I argue that disability education is vitally important for a truly modern world. We can't claim to be something we're not, that's unfair for everyone, as things like this deserve to be highlighted. Enough with the stereotyping. It's 2024 as of writing this. We are supposed to be an equal opportunities society, but we aren't. We claim to be, but really, how can we be? You can't have your cake and eat it too. If we educate children, notably in PSHE sessions, in time (as it will take time) there's no escaping this fact. There's no 'quick fix', but if we stick with it, hopefully disability will get the respect it deserves.

After all, ...

"Knowledge is power' – [Francis Bacon]

If disability education is implemented, then there's a chance of mental health deterioration lowering significantly. The more people learn the truth about disability, the more likelihood of acceptance. I discussed in *Disabling Ableism* that PSHE lessons would be the perfect opportunity to educate about disabilities as these lessons are purposely designed to teach about life. The *Department of Education (DoE)* and the *Education Workforce Council (EWC)* are missing a trick with the PSHE lessons. These lessons are perfect to educate about disabilities. I've actually decided to contact these departments to ask the question. Watch this space.

It does make a lot of sense. Disability is a part of society, that's the reality, so why isn't the topic spoken about openly? If it's a case of being terrified of saying the wrong thing, then people shouldn't have to be fearful. Questions are good. That's how we learn. Again, I think I said this before, but I've experienced people avoiding me, speaking to my parents instead of speaking to me, and one instance that still stays with me happened a few years ago. A mother and child were walking down the street one day, and I was driving down the opposite way, when I suddenly hear the child asking the mother, *"Mum, what's wrong with that girl? Why is she in a wheelchair?"* Now, this is absolutely fine with me, I'd rather be asked questions, especially if it's a child. Children are inquisitive. Asking questions are how children learn about the different things around them, about the world. The mother just rushed the child along and told them not to stare. This reaction to a genuine question was what I took issue with. Children mean no harm, they ask because they want to know, and I'm always more than happy to answer if it means that disability education will be at the forefront of the conversation. Something that isn't as well-known as it should be. Avoiding only creates more unanswered questions.

It says a lot that we are so open about a wide variety of topics, but one specific topic, there's radio silence. The shutters automatically come down when topics considered 'difficult' are spoken about. Nobody wants to know, and that's sad and disappointing.

However, one school I know of for a fact doesn't shy away from the topic of disability, they embrace it. This particular school acknowledges disability awareness, which I'm extremely pleased with. This is what is needed. How do I know about the acknowledgement? It's Tommy's school.

The Education Debate

As a reminder, Tommy is my nephew who is in primary school to put it into context.

Recently, Tommy had to dress in green to acknowledge *World Cerebral Palsy Awareness Day,* which is on 6th October annually, which is perfect. Teaching the curriculum is important, but everyday topics, such as disability is equally as important to teach. Children are the future, let's teach about disability awareness and equality. This is what matters.

In short, disability education is vital. Now, I said before that DoE, EWC and education in general should be showing an interest in delivering and also learning about disability, well recently, my publisher Allan and I had the wonderful opportunity to give talks in educational establishments, in *Coleg Cambria* and *Wrexham University* respectively. This shows positive progression.

We gave the talks to students in *Wrexham University* and staff and students in *Coleg Cambria*. It really was a successful experience. Both students and staff alike were very enthusiastic and interested in the subject matter in both establishments, which really makes a difference meeting people who are actually genuinely interested in the subject matter, and how they can help to improve disability equality. It's refreshing for me personally, as I have come up against some much backlash in the past just because of my physical appearance. I know that these talks had the desired impact because I had such extremely positive feedback after. When I know people are genuinely interested, it makes my job a whole lot easier. What I found baffling though is that students in *Wrexham University* knew of the term 'ableism', whereas staff at *Coleg Cambria* wasn't aware of the term at all. To be honest, I wasn't aware of the term's 'ableism' and 'ableist' either before writing *Disabling Ableism*. Maybe it's because students are more technology focused, and the terms are relatively new? Well, I would come to that conclusion, but...

"The term was coined by US feminists in the 1980s and was later used by the Council of the London Borough of Haringey in a press release in 1986." – ['Ableism', Oxford reference.com]

The Education Debate

So, I really don't know why some people know of this term, whereas others don't. Ignorance? Fear? Who knows?

All staff at educational establishments **need** to recognise and understand the terms 'ableism' and 'ableist', and the attitude it brings, in order to help eradicate it for the future generations. Saying that however, during the staff talk at *Coleg Cambria*, one staff member cautiously gave their answer to what the terms meant, (their answer was correct by the way), but this reaction goes to prove that people are fearful of giving the wrong answer in case they offend a person with a disability. This fear is offensive, because nobody talks about disability in the way it should be discussed, it opens up a danger of mental health deterioration. Does this make sense? When Allan asked my opening question in my speech, what disability means, again there was an apprehension there, again probably because of the fear of offending. Everyone should have a basic idea of disability, right? The staff members actually did have the basic idea at a fundamental level, it became much harder when

Allan asked if they knew what disability actually meant. The overall consensus was that it was a much more difficult question. One staff member said that it depends on the person who has a disability. This is exactly what it means. There's not one answer, there are many answers depending on the person, but ultimately the disability itself should never overshadow the person. That's the long and short of it. It was the same with the students at *Wrexham University*, you could sense the fear of answering both questions. The looks of genuine fear in that moment were palpable. In those moments, I saw the fear of society in real time. It was an interesting experiment to say the least.

Educators are in a perfect position to educate the right topics. Another staff member said during the talk, that the staff at the college only have a basic understanding of a new student's needs when they first begin college life, and so, only have so many resources to work with, and as a result, can only do so much, which is absolutely gut-wrenching for me. The college asked my publisher Allan and I to give these talks, were really, local Government should be the ones to provide staff training. It shouldn't be up to educational establishments to arrange talks of this nature. The Department of Education should make disability awareness a part of staff training days.

There again, for this to have any kind of success, involving those with disabilities to come and train local Government on how to deliver effective training that will help educational establishments will work wonders for disability equality. Going in without any **actual** training, (and by actual training I mean, involving people with lived experience, and not just going off assumptions). It's those assumptions that ultimately cause mental health issues for people with disabilities. You are only giving a surface level teaching otherwise, more than likely, misinformation from the Internet. In order to give a true teaching that will make the desired impact, you **need to involve those with disabilities**, plain and simple, otherwise, what's the point?

A genuine want to end ableism and not just do it as a tick box exercise will ultimately work wonders on not only disability equality but can also have a positive impact on mental health, as it's all interconnected.

Education VS. Work

Earlier, I spoke about social fear of disability and how this can play a part in attitudes. I wholeheartedly believe if disability education was part of the curriculum and a part of training in work, then we would see half of the blatant ableism today. Awareness and action begins at ground level.

There seems to be an ignorance currently when education prepare pupils for the world of work, especially pupils with disabilities. I know this because it's something that I've personally experienced.

When I was 16 in secondary school, pupils from my year group (including myself) had mock job interviews, where people from the Education Department would come into school to act as an interviewer and give the pupils tips on how to improve their interview skills. This is great, and

The Education Debate

great for me, because the person who was 'interviewing' me told me that I was perfect. I was confident, clear, kept eye-contact, polite, etc., etc., but this only ultimately set me up to fail.

This wasn't the reality. I really do wish I knew the reality back then, as I may have been better equipped to deal with such ableism in the world of work.

Nobody during this time, took me to one side and warned me about the difficulties I would potentially face from potential employers because of my mild Cerebral Palsy. It gave me false hope. I was unprepared. Yes, the truth would've hurt, and yes, there's an argument to be made that explaining this to me may have exasperated my mental health issues, but to counteract this, it could've been the making of me from the very beginning.

School prepares you for work, but work **isn't** prepared for you, and this is only the tip of the iceberg for disability and society in general.

Chapter 14
What Disability Actually Means to Us

This, in all honesty is a very difficult thing to give a clear answer to. You see, disability isn't just one thing, (although society likes to think it is, in order to put it into a box, and not have to deal with the different iterations of the subject). During mine and Allan's recent talks in educational establishments, it was actually during the staff training talk we delivered in the college, I asked in the speech, does anyone know what disability actually means? After a long pause, one staff member reluctantly raised their hand and said that it depends on the individual. This is exactly right. Not all disabilities are the same, so it shouldn't be treated as the same. It's crucially important to note that people's disabilities can be mild, moderate or severe, but yet again, whatever the severity of said disability, that doesn't mean, nor does it give you the right to treat us any differently from the next person.

What Disability Actually Means to Us

Some people identify as having a disability, whereas, like me, others don't. That's not to say we're delusional, we just choose not to be defined as this one image. The title of my first book indicated this exact fact. A picture paints a thousand words. A label paints a million more. The disability label often only paints a million negative words in the eyes of society, this is why people who have disabilities tend to distance away from the term. The word itself is negative. Distancing ourselves from the term is an attempt to maintain our mental health, but it is difficult, given the situation we find ourselves in. What society needs to understand and accept is that disability is individual to the person, and how we decide to live is up to us, if we are capable of making the choice. Note, I said live, not exist. Often we are treated as just as existing. We're not allowed to live as we intend to. Society does like to patronise and gas-light people with disabilities into thinking that we're in control of our own lives, whereas really, it's society who are pulling the strings like a secret puppet master. This mistreatment obviously lends itself to developing potential mental health issues.

According to the *Disability Equality Act of 2010:*

"You're disabled under the Equality Act 2010 if you have a physical or mental impairment that has a 'substantial' and 'long-term' negative effect on your ability to do normal daily activities." – [Definition of disability under the Equality Act 2010', Gov.UK].

The Government's choice of wording in this quote I take issue with. Negative and normal. Everything is negative. Furthermore, what's a normal everyday task? This quote just screams ableism all on it's own. Saying 'normal' only exasperates the issue. This implies that disability isn't 'normal', (or a standard part of life as I like to refer to it), thus creating further hidden barriers which can be damaging to repairing the relationship between society and disability. This language only plays into the stereotype. Our abilities are individual (I feel like a broken record), so who's to say that a non-disabled person may experience days where their

What Disability Actually Means to Us

capabilities may not be up to par? Saying that only a person with a disability can have negative experiences which can impact negatively on the person's ability to do everyday tasks is abhorrent. Where's the evidence? Unless you have tangible proof, then this is just scaremongering, and therefore disgusting.

I've said before that I know I'm disabled, it's obvious, but I choose not to be reminded of it by identifying as the label. I don't see myself as disabled. I see myself as Sam and that's it, or auntie Sam when I'm with Rosie and Tommy. I'm going on a slight tangent here, but I'm so glad that I started my writing career. Rosie read *CP Isn't Me* when it was first published back in 2022, and it did save a lot of awkward questions on her part I feel. She now knows absolutely everything about me, what I went through and how it affected me as a person. She's hopefully become more aware of the struggles a person with a disability faces every single day of their lives, and feels confident enough to call it out when she sees it. I'm not blowing my own trumpet here, but there was a time during her younger years that Rosie wouldn't look at me. I feel that the chair made her uncomfortable as she didn't understand why I had to use a wheelchair. As soon as she read *CP Isn't Me*, those initial fears went away. She truly understands now, and she's like my best friend now. She's always looking out for me, and I truly appreciate that. Giving children the opportunity to learn and understand about disability is no mean feat. I believe it's necessary. To go from not being looked at to constantly being by my side says something for disability education.

The thing is, every single person on the planet has different abilities, whether you're disabled or otherwise. It can be argued that your capabilities can have a negative effect on your ability to do daily activities regardless of who you are. It's dependent on the person. Nobody is superhuman. I also take issue with the 'normal' description that the Government website has chosen to use here. What is a 'normal' daily activity? This word alone can make a person with a disability of some form feel worthless and incapable right off the bat. It gives society the false narrative. It feeds into the

What Disability Actually Means to Us

stereotype. This is just **1** example of how a word can create a perception that is completely false. I completely understand that there are some things that people with a disability may find a little more difficult to execute, but to outright say that if you have a disability, you are unable to do general tasks is abhorrent. This type of blanketing isn't necessary. It shouldn't be a thing. People in power should be aware of how their words can have a negative impact on not only a person with a disability, but general society as a whole. A single phrase, sentence or even a single word can have devastating consequences on those who are considered to be the main target.

I recently (as of writing this) had the privilege of attending *Wrexham University* to deliver a talk to students on disability awareness and equality, alongside my publisher Allan. During the Q&A session following the speech, a student gave a very interesting, and insightful outlook. The 2nd person may I add, in as many months to make this exact same observation.

What Disability Actually Means to Us

"You aren't disabled, it's society that actually disables you." – [Student From Wrexham University]

Again, I wholeheartedly agree. It's so interesting to me that this is the 2nd time I've heard this, from 2 separate people in general society who have no connection to each other whatsoever. It is telling though that there is awareness in a small capacity at least that the issue exists and it's mainly due to public perceptions. It gives me hope of future equal opportunities for all, but my hope is extremely slim line however unfortunately, as in reality, I know that equality for all won't come to full fruition. I hope society will eventually change my mind. I'm willing society to look at the subject of disability and subsequent mental health issues and rethink their beliefs.

The terms 'disabled' and 'disability' are supposed to be descriptive words, which is absolutely fine. I have said in the past that I hate those terms, but this hatred materialised as soon as I was only known for having a disability. I disappeared. Faded away. A label replacing me. The person. My hatred started

What Disability Actually Means to Us

as soon as I began secondary school, (which by now, is well documented), and lasted until I was well into my mid-to-late twenties. I never had any issues with my Cerebral Palsy before secondary school, I had no reason to. I was treated as a child, not a disabled child, obviously I was, but the disability label didn't become my identity until I eventually reached the age of 11. When I was in the midst of this hatred, I found myself longing for the days where my disability didn't matter to anyone. I didn't feel stigmatised as a child, so this sudden change in attitude was a shock for me, to say the least.

Disability shouldn't be the be all and end all of a person. Disability should be a part of us, not the whole package.

This form of rejection can ultimately become a serious issue as soon as the rejection affects your mental health. What society **needs** to understand and accept is that you can have a disability, but you may not identify yourself as disabled. Your disability maybe obvious or not, but whatever your form of disability, which shouldn't mean you have to identify yourself as disabled. You're a person first, a disability second. This is extremely important to understand and accept. The lecturer at *Wrexham University* when I attended for the speech, said that they had a previous student with a disability who didn't want to be labelled as 'disabled' and who gave an impassioned speech not to identify them as that. They despised the term. It's a label. A negative prefix that society becomes obsessed with strangely. This obsession with disabilities and labelling only makes mental health worse. We are only one dimensional in society's eyes. Its enforcement on us, that label. A label which is so redundant in comparison to other, more important and pressing issues the world has to contend with every single day of our lives. It really doesn't matter.

We don't impose our beliefs on other demographics, but disability does seem to have been forced into this bullying corner. All of society's misplaced anger and judgement seems to be squarely placed on this one demographic. It's because disability isn't as widely known and recognised to general society, as the topic isn't as intergraded into today's society as it should be. Disability has no respect whatsoever. Disability is just a word, not a lifestyle. Yes, we live our lives as best we can as a person with a disability, but we generally don't define ourselves as disabled. Trying to get this important message across to the public is extremely difficult. We must keep fighting if we want equality which could be seen as counterintuitive, but it's true.

This is the issue, disability doesn't always mean inability, but society somehow continues to make that connection. This is what I mean, just in case there was any confusion by the statement.

The terms 'disability' and 'disabled' should only be used when it is necessary, such as, booking tickets for events, (in order to make sure that your accessibility requirements are properly met), or medical reasons, education enrolment, any type of formality really, but it shouldn't be used to describe a person in everyday scenarios, especially in a negative way, which somehow today, the terms almost, always are used in a negative way. There's

What Disability Actually Means to Us

absolutely no rhyme or reason to do so. What is the benefit, other than to only cause added distress to the person in question?

We are more than our disabilities.

Chapter 15
Conclusion

In a strange way, I guess I'm grateful for the mistreatment I have faced. Don't get me wrong, it was an agonising experience, something of which I wouldn't wish on anyone, but if I didn't have those negative experiences, my mental health wouldn't have deteriorated to the point where I eventually thought that I'd try to write a book. It is funny how life turns out; I didn't think for one minute that I'd be an author. I had ambitions of being a graphic designer and that was it. That's what I wanted to do with my life. After all, I studied, and eventually graduated in graphic design. I love designing and creating. This was the profession I thought I was going to strive in. Little did I know that society wouldn't provide me with the opportunity really. I wasn't prepared for the denial. This was a constant and literal fight, a fight that I wasn't prepared for. The cold, hard truth is that employers have a problem with hiring people with disabilities and come up with a number of excuses not to hire a

Conclusion

person with a disability, which are based on assumptions. This is 2024 soon to be 2025, are we still going to carry on with this farcical approach to disability?

If people were willing to teach and learn the truth about disability, I feel this obviously would help to eventually eradicate ableism, and mental health issues as an extension. Unfortunately, though, this doesn't seem to be the case. Due to this constant ignorance which negatively impacted me mentally, I reached a stage where I thought enough was enough. I took up Ceri's suggestion. I had to try something. I needed an outlet. An escape from the reality I existed in.

Yes, I was always encouraged by my dad, my English teacher in secondary school and eventually years later, my sister-in-law Ceri to write, but at that early point in my life, it didn't interest me at all. Being creative did. I understand now that writing is a form of creativity, a creativeness which can also have a great, and positive impact on not only yourself, but also the reader. It can have the power to change perceptions.

Conclusion

For me, writing has been tremendously beneficial to my mental health. It's cathartic, it's a form of therapy which I can go to whenever I want. If you're struggling, believe me, just try it. Try writing everything down that's plaguing your mind. At first, I didn't believe writing would work, but believe me, it definitely does. Yes, I've officially become an author as a result, but this is just my story, you can just write everything down privately if you prefer. Trust me, it will be a great weight lifted.

I also thought that nobody would be interested in my writing when dad and my English teacher tried to encourage me down this path, and besides, what was I going to write about? I thought I had no material, no subject on which to write a book. Little did I know that I had the material. I was living it.

Mental health decline can blur you from what you have, from what you are, and what you could be. It's debilitating. You have a little voice in your head telling you that you're a failure, and you will always be a failure no matter what you try to do. Having any disability confirms this in the eyes of society at least. You are constantly rejected, patronised,

Conclusion

stigmatised, segregated. In a way, it is like living back in the years 1948-1994 where Apartheid ruled. Maybe not in the exact same way, but in silence. Under the surface. Invisible. You can't blatantly see it, but it's there. It's just the disability version.

You are judged and ridiculed constantly. You are made to feel inadequate to the next person who doesn't have a disability, but to counteract this, we are also inspiring, strong and brave. A very obvious contradiction when written down. It's confusing. Which are we? We can't be both, but neither do we want to be. Labels are the things that we need to distance ourselves away from, not encourage.

It really does annoy me, because we are just expected to be grateful for what we do have (which **is** minimal) and accept the mistreatment.

"I feel it's important that we shine a light on the mental health impact of lifelong disability. There's a lot of pressure out there to be the 'cheery' disabled person but we're human like everyone else!" – [Richard Luke, Specialist

Conclusion

Information Officer and Cerebral Palsy Programme Lead, Scope]

I hope you can understand by now the mental implications this rejection can have. The expectation of having a constant 'cheery' and grateful attitude can be draining. We are expected just to know our place in society, and be okay with it? This doesn't fly in the 'modern' 21st century. This attitude is Dickensian and should never have been allowed to happen throughout humanity, throughout history, but personally I think that it's gotten worse somehow, as soon as this 'modern' concept was introduced ironically.

I remember in secondary school, being told by a support worker, of all people, that I should be grateful for having a mild disability, compared to someone they knew who had a severe disability. This is a clear ableist attitude, something that shouldn't happen in the 21st century. Comparison is wrong, it gives people complexes which in turn, can severely damage our mental health. Yes, the incident happened in 2004, but this outdated attitude is something that should have already

Conclusion

been abolished, but it still truly hasn't. Disability awareness has missed the train when it comes to disability equality and inclusion.

However, disability awareness is starting to gain momentum today, but disability is far from where it should be in society given the 'modern world'. Other topics that are deemed important to be recognised by society are race, sexual orientation, and transgressions to give a few examples. My issue with this is that disability isn't nearly as important as other subjects. I would argue that there is a tier system which society either knowingly or unknowingly actively helps to create this ableism we have (as a society) have become immune to. It's just extremely sad.

Comparing disabilities doesn't work anyway, it shouldn't matter the form of our disabilities, we should, and deserve to be treated the same as each other, but recognising our strengths and rewarding those strengths, and not out of sympathy or empathy, but our true characteristics, alongside the rest of the population, and when I say the 'same', I mean the same opportunities. There's an argument to be made that saying 'the same' can be discriminate in itself, as people are individual and have different abilities that deserve to be respected. For any hope of rebuilding disability relations with society in general, there needs to be genuine understanding, acceptance and action. It's not enough just to say something. You need to start doing something which will ultimately help repair the relationship in the future.

There should **never** be a hierarchy of any demographic whatsoever. Nobody is superior to anyone else. A severely disabled person still has a personality. Their ways of communication maybe a little different, but their life should never be judged by appearance alone, and instantly put on a lower tier to a person with a moderate or mild disability. This attitude is wrong on so many levels. It's actually disgusting. This attitude can create so many issues related to mental health, but this isn't acknowledged because disability isn't acknowledged in the way it should be. Mental health decline becomes as ignored as disability is, when it's actually a person with a disability who is

Conclusion

experiencing the mental health deterioration. Mental health issues fade away with how much the disability dominates. This though, potentially only creates further mental health deterioration, which is a vicious cycle.

The pressure that it must undertake to actually claim to be a 'modern' society must be immense and daunting. There's bound to be something that will inevitably slip through the cracks. Rightly, I feel that society is slowly working on their attitudes towards racism and homophobia the most, which is extremely encouraging. To me, it just goes to show that society is capable of going the extra mile to understand these important topics, arguably to the point of obsession, as a means to rectify the misconceptions these types of topics pose. However, if you do only concentrate on certain demographics, then it's inevitable that ableism for example, will fall by the wayside in terms of importance. I think it is quite telling the state of disability if Richard Luke from *Scope* is saying that people with disabilities are expected to be 'cheery' in the face of adversity. It just goes to show, (in my mind at least), actually how much needs to be done to improve disability relations. A human being cannot be expected to be 'cheery' 24/7, it's unhealthy. Contrary to popular belief, people with disabilities, (whatever it be), are in fact human beings at the end of the day, as Richard has said.

If there was this type of rejection in general society, I can well imagine that something would be done quickly to try and rectify it. A person with a disability doesn't have that option. You've read about how this negativity can have detrimental effects on others who have a disability. Dehumanizing. This is one word that sticks out, because you do feel dehumanized and useless, as if all of your achievements count for nothing. This is how I felt anyway. You start thinking back to when you were bullied and think that those bullies were right in what they said. For me, it was that I'd never amount to much, nobody wants me, nobody loves me, you're alone and always will be alone, you're a burden. Why don't you just kill yourself? Nobody would miss you anyway. Those thoughts return tenfold when mental health deterioration starts.

Conclusion

Personally, I began to believe what those bullies said. After all, nobody wanted me, that's what I thought at the time anyway.

I really have trouble believing that people actually understand how their words and/or actions may affect any person. You don't know what they have gone through, or indeed, are going through, especially as a person with a disability of some kind. Yes, you may show empathy for the person, but you don't know what it's really like, trying to navigate through life where the society is just full of hate. Your words and/or actions have more impact, more influence than you may think.

What we need to do is stop denying people, especially those who have a disability, and encourage them, respect them, by opening up those opportunities and making public places fully accessible. We need to start being welcoming. If a person with a disability isn't the right candidate for a job, based on their skills alone, that's fine, but never deny us solely on our disabilities. This behaviour is ableist, immoral and unethical to say the least.

When I started my 1st volunteering job after graduating, I had a support worker who accompanied me to work, where they also supported others. One client was severely disabled which is absolutely fine, but the support worker at the time said to **me** that the other client's family should end this client's life. Why? Well, because the client couldn't do anything in the support worker's opinion. Every life is precious. I obviously was horrified when the support worker said this to me. Not only is it abhorrent to say, but it's also an invasion of privacy. A support worker should never discuss clients openly, this is unprofessional and immoral. It's ethically corrupt.

Every person deserves respect, something that the support worker at the time didn't give to the other person.

It just gave me food for thought, realising that disability isn't respected at all, even with some (not all) in the care profession.

"Showing people respect removes barriers that often affect people with CP. This helps them

Conclusion

successfully cope with mental health issues. People with a disability can enjoy good mental health with proper assessment and support." – *[Counsellor Beryl Blackmore, Wrexham Mayor 2024-2025]*

Society is so keen nowadays to help end the stigma of mental health, but for a person with a disability, it is pointless as the stigma of disability continues to grow. Society may say that they are accepting of everyone whatever their background, but obviously, there's still a long way to go. If society was accepting, then my books would be redundant, people with disabilities and mental health wouldn't feel the need to speak out about their personal experiences and opinions, and how this treatment, (or indeed, mistreatment) go onto affect the person's mental health. Unfortunately, though, this is a common occurrence.

To truly help end the stigma of mental health, we first need to end the stigma around the things that can contribute to potential mental health decline, including the negative perceptions of disability. We're punished for having a disability, imprisoned actually. I know that life isn't fair, but come on, still treating people like enemy no. 1 over something that we cannot control, is evil and should be addressed and eradicated immediately.

For the benefit of this book, ending the stigma around disability is a fantastic starting point. There also needs to be proper assessment and support available as the Mayor of Wrexham from 2024-2025, Counsellor Beryl Blackmore said.

I personally have tried counselling, but I think because my mental health issues were quite unique as they revolved mostly around my Cerebral Palsy, and not being given the same opportunities as the rest of society, the counselling wasn't equipped to deal with such specific issues, and so, as a result, my experience of attending counselling wasn't the best. It ultimately just made me feel worse, and I realised that counselling really is a 'one size fits all' approach. It wasn't tailored to any specific type of mental health issue. The treatments were the same in my eyes. As a result, I just felt like another patient. When you're dealing with mental health issues, the last thing you need is to feel like just

Conclusion

another patient. You need techniques and advice specific to you and your situation.

As the years have rolled by, I've realised that the only person who I can truly trust is myself, and of course, my family. People come and go, they may say things for you to feel included, but really, they are only doing it for their own ends. At the end of the day, people are only interested in one thing, themselves. This is what I've come to realise. Yes, it may sound harsh, and a bit pessimistic, something which I think you weren't expecting to read in a book like this. Depending on others to make you happy, never works, only you can do that.

It does make being seen for who you are more difficult if you have a disability of some kind, but never mistake patronisation for kindness. Never give others the satisfaction of being the one you turn to for reassurance, only family, and good friends can do that. Others only see you as weak and play on that weakness. In my case, especially for one example, some people played with my emotions constantly. I went to them at a very dark period of my life. The best way I can describe these people are wolves in sheep clothing. They thought I was weak because of the disability yes, but also because of the added trauma I experienced up to that point. I ended up relying on these people. It was like a form of coercive control. These people used to be around me one minute and gone the next. They liked to play mind games, and I was so far gone mentally, that I couldn't see what was happening, I was devoted to them. Again, I've decided not to go into the specifics of the mistreatment as I covered it in *CP Isn't Me*. All I will say is that the mistreatment destroyed any little self-respect and self-esteem I had left. By the end I was a crumbling mess.

I consider myself quite lucky now in terms of having a platform which allows me to finally speak out on disability injustices. My outlook however may seem cynical, and you may come to the conclusion that I'm not actually happy because I still have trust issues, given what I've just said, but in actuality, I am happy. I'm optimistic about life, because I'm determined not to be mistreated again. This career has helped me to understand this. I'm feeling more

Conclusion

confident in myself, I've now had my nose pierced, (something that I didn't think I could ever do, because I was scared of not being liked), from the mistreatment I faced during my life, I came to the conclusion a long time ago that nobody actually likes me anyway, so why don't I do something that would make me happy and confident for a change? Trying to please others was only making me miserable. I had it done really to say to people that this is me, I'm happy, I'm confident, and if you don't like it, you know what to do. I'm so tired of trying to please others. My piercings (ears and nose) also are a symbol of defiance. I like to think it sends a message to society that people with disabilities can have piercings too, alongside so many other mundane things, thus quashing the stereotype.

I've also had a new voluntary job as a Tenancy Support Officer and Social Media Developer for a care company which specialises in adapting houses for people with disabilities to live as independently as possible. My new boss is lovely, and I feel they have my best intentions at heart. My new voluntary work genuinely appreciates me, I'm treated extremely well. This job has come around since I started my writing career. One thing leads to another. I have a lot to thank becoming an author for, and in turn, my immediate family, (mum, dad, Ian, Ceri, Rosie, Tommy, my late nan Mary, even my late dog Bubbles), for supporting me throughout, even though the tough times. Thank you so much to my dad, and my sister-in-law, Ceri for pushing me to begin writing. Thank you to my extended family, (my uncle Alfie and cousins) for supporting me by attending the book launches and loving me for who I am, not what I am. I truly appreciate it.

Thank you so much to my publisher Allan for kindly agreeing to publish my books. Your acceptance kicked off a brighter outlook on life for me after being in such a dark place for so many years. I'll always be grateful for that.

Finally, thank you ever so much to each and every single person who I've had the privilege to meet, interact and work with. Without your support, my books wouldn't be known.

Conclusion

So yes, I am happy, I've discovered myself again, I've gone passed caring of what people think of me. I'm stronger now, but for so many others though, it is like fighting a losing battle. All we want is to be treated the same way as everyone else in society, (and this goes for all types of disabilities – mild, moderate and severe). News flash, we are all human at the end of the day with personalities and opinions. This second-class citizen approach is so outdated, and so damaging to mental health. For one example, I understand that there are those who are unable to speak, but this doesn't mean that they're any less than the next non-disabled person.

We deserve to have equality and diversity. This is what makes a democracy at the end of the day. Treatment of disability, as it currently stands is bewildering to me. A disability of any kind should never be judged. Who are you to make that judgement? We all breathe, eat, sleep, bleed, use a bathroom. Why should we be seen and treated as 'different' from people who don't know us from Adam? How is this fair? I think because disability has a reputation for being 'vulnerable' and 'different', society may believe that it then gives them permission to empathise and/or patronise. You don't know us; you haven't lived our lives. Yet, you have given yourself permission to pretend to know 'what we're going through'? How? I can 100% guarantee you cannot identify yourself with us, or even understand what we deal with daily. You probably wouldn't survive in all honesty. You are only putting your perceptions onto us, which can have severe negative consequences to our mental health in the long term. This is so important to establish, understand, accept, and stop. You may feel as if you are being considerate, but you are really doing more harm than good in all honesty. Please don't put us on a pedestal, nor disown us, we aren't your pet to 'look after' or play games with. We are **real** human beings who have **real** feelings. Our disabilities are secondary to us. Our disabilities are just one aspect of us, just like eye colours, hair colours, a disability should never be the be all and end all of a person. It's absolutely ridiculous that we still highlight disability as a negative. It's neither negative or positive. A

Conclusion

disability is just that, a disability. Making it the prominent feature of a person is Dickensian and Orwellian at the same time. We take everything at face value and are willing to accept the 1st thing we're told about something. It seems that we cannot form our own opinions anymore as we rely too heavily on technology to tell us what to do and believe, which should go without saying, has a whole host of different negatives on the entire population generally. This reliance only creates further mental anguish to others in society, sometimes through no fault of their own, technology has a firm grip on us that it can be extremely difficult to trust other **viable** sources of information. It is to go with our fast paced lifestyle we have today. You would have to put the work in to find information related to a certain topic, this is where the Internet is the preferred option where sensationalism rules, which unfortunately is at the cost of one's own mental health deterioration.

For the next two paragraphs, I'm going to talk to each and every single person with a disability of some kind, alongside society as a whole.

Conclusion

I'm talking to you now, the person who has a disability. I'm not going to lie, things are bleak for a person with a disability. There's so much discrimination and so many assumptions associated with disability, it can be extremely difficult to see the light at the end of the tunnel. Believe me, I can definitely attest to this unfortunately.

These things though should never have any bearing on you as a person. When someone says "no", (believe me, you'll come across individuals who are still living in the dark ages with disabilities, because this is what will happen). I can unfortunately guarantee you that. When those things do happen, be defiant. Keep saying "yes you can" until someone listens. You may get tired of defending yourself constantly, but you will get there. It may not seem like it now, but continue with the fight. You'll eventually be recognised and respected by the **whole of society** if you keep going. This is when the *'Keep Calm and Carry On'* phrase is crucial. Regardless of the severity of your disability and mental health issue, I'm going to say

Conclusion

something now that I've learned since becoming an author.

Never be afraid to just be yourself. Never be afraid to question 'authority'. If you ask questions, you are showing that you're strong willed and understand when you're being discriminated against. This is when the tables will turn. You'll receive respect and in some cases, equality. Asking questions as to why a certain thing is designed that way, or why you're being treated differently to the rest of society, will really open the floor for real positive change to happen. Defiance is the best tool at your disposal. Say "no" to mistreatment, "no" to stereotyping, "no" to issues with mental health due to public perceptions which are outdated, offensive and false. I'm saying this as someone who questioned the system and as a result, is gaining more respect and responsibility. Challenge the system, instead of it challenging you.

Determination will ultimately get you noticed for who you are, rather than what you are. Once that happens, you will then have the pleasure of showing off your worth to those who doubted you, not bragging, but letting people know that they were wrong to doubt you, by doing this, I have no doubt in my mind that issues with mental health will decrease fir those with disabilities. It worked for me. Of course, you'll suffer defeats in life, everyone does, regardless of who they are, the key is not let the negatives define you as a person. You're worth so much more.

I also just want to say that it's good to cry every now and then. It's therapeutic. Never bottle things up, otherwise when those feelings erupt, they truly erupt. A good cry resets you to be stronger. Mental health issues will pass in time, with the right support, mainly I've found from people who know you, like family and friends. Without my family during that dark period of my life, I dread to think what could've happened. If family and friends aren't an option, then contacting mental health charities such as The Samaritans and is are out there. The correct support is important.

Lesley Griffiths, Member of the Senedd for Wrexham has also kindly given vital information where you can get support if needed.

Conclusion

"There are a number of organisations and charities, such as Mind Cymru and the C.A.L.L. mental health helpline. Another significant breakthrough in recent times has been the introduction of the NHS 111 'Press 2' service, which offers urgent mental health support to people of all ages and abilities across Wales, 24 hours a day, seven days a week. In October 2024, the Royal College of Psychiatrists completed a review of the first year of the implementation. Approximately 120,000 calls were received in the first 12 months, and 99 per cent of those calls during the review period led to a reduction in distress, with individuals being provided with a compassionate and timely response." – [Lesley Griffiths, Member of the Senedd for Wrexham]

To society, please never judge a book by its cover. You don't know what a person with a disability could be going through. Carelessness and ableism can cause serious issues mentally, physically and emotionally. Why do you want to be the cause of further mental health deterioration? Our *NHS* is struggling as it is, without ableism being yet another issue. All we're asking for is proper understanding and action to help drive the point across. Judging others from appearance alone is wrong. Be the generation to nip ableism and by extension, mental health issues in the bush for good. We owe it to each other.

To finish, I would like to add a quote from Lesley Griffiths, Member of the Senedd for Wrexham:

"It is by no means an easy task, but I hope there are signs of promise, and we are heading in the right direction. If anyone is struggling or if you're concerned for the wellbeing of a friend or loved one, support is available and talking to someone can make a world of difference." – [Lesley Griffiths, Member of the Senedd for Wrexham]

As Lesley Griffiths MS for Wrexham mentioned, there is help available if you or a loved one is struggling, which is good to know that there's help readily available if needed, but really, unless we start to tackle ableism in all its forms ourselves,

Conclusion

mental health issues are still going to remain. To truly end mental health deterioration, we must dig out the root causes. I keep saying it, but I truly believe that education is a good place to start, it's not the only answer by any means, but education is a great place to start the eradication of ableism. Then, and only then, can we start to see a true end to mental health issues. Thus, potentially ending the...

Silence.

Thank you

Publisher

J. Allan Longshadow

Book Cover Artwork Artist

Martin Maxwell

Participants

Lesley Griffiths, Member of the Senedd for Wrexham

Counsellor Beryl Blackmore, Wrexham Mayor 2024 - 2025

Conclusion

Richard Luke, Specialist Information Officer and Cerebral Palsy Programme Lead, Scope

Jeff Dawson, CEO of 1st Enable Ltd.

Jayne Knight, Ling Trust

Annette Cmela, Global Chief Brand Officer, Hidden Disabilities Sunflower

Chantal Boyle, Communications Manager, Hidden Disabilities Sunflower

Dr. Frances Ryan, Guardian columnist and journalist, author

'Diz', social media participant

Rachel Williams, social media participant

Ben Ashby, social media participant

Rebekah Sims, social media participant

Ian Jarvis, social media participant

Jasper Colquhon, social media participant

John Pam Lloreda, social media participant

'Jme' Elias, social media participant

Conclusion

Organisations

Mind

Sense

Scope

Hidden Disabilities Sunflower

1st Enable Ltd.

Ling Trust

House of Lords Library, London

House of Commons Library, London

NHS (National Health Service)

Family

Mum

Dad

Ian

Ceri

Rosie

Tommy

Conclusion

My late nan, Mary

My late dog, Bubbles

I know I've said this at the beginning of this book, but thank you to you, the reader for taking the time to read not only this book, but hopefully every book I've written up to this point. Without your continued support and interest, I wouldn't be who I am today.

In an ideal world, highlighting disability awareness and equality wouldn't have to happen as it would be commonplace. Equality is obvious today. It's recognised...to a point.

Disability equality should have the same level of awareness, just as race, gender, sexual orientation just to name a few, and by reading my books, you are helping with the fight to end the stigma of disability, and by extension mental health issues related to disability.

I hope you take something from my books, something that you will help advocate for, and not

Conclusion

just to read, place on a shelf, then forget. I hope you will act and help me in my personal mission to end discrimination for all, and yes, this definitely, and especially includes ableism.

Now is the time to end ableism for the future generations.

A Sneak Peak: Future Plans

My next project is going to be for children which will involve my fantastic nephew, Tommy. Thank you, Tommy, for being involved in this next important project.

My lovely niece, Rosie, has kindly agreed to illustrate this next important project. Thank you, Rosie, I look forward to working alongside you.

This next project aims to highlight not only Cerebral Palsy, but also other disabilities to the younger generation, in the hopes of eliminating ableism for the future.

SAMANTHA MAXWELL'S BOOK LIST AS OF SEPTEMBER 2025:

CP Isn't Me – Released December 2022

Disabling Ableism – Released April 2024

SILENCED. – Released September 2025

Printed in Dunstable, United Kingdom

72394425R00201